MW00930843

MEDICAL QIGONG EXERCISE PRESCRIPTIONS

MEDICAL QIGONG EXERCISE PRESCRIPTIONS

A Self-Healing Guide for Patients & Practitioners

Suzanne B. Friedman, L.Ac., DMQ (China)

Copyright © 2006 by Suzanne B. Friedman, L.Ac., DMQ (China).

Library of Congress Number: 2006900377
ISBN :   Hardcover   1-4257-0715-7
                  Softcover   1-4257-0714-9

All rights reserved. No part of this book may be reproduced or transmitted in any form or by any means, electronic or mechanical, including photocopying, recording, or by any information storage and retrieval system, without permission in writing from the copyright owner.

This book was printed in the United States of America.

To order additional copies of this book, contact:
Xlibris Corporation
1-888-795-4274
www.Xlibris.com
Orders@Xlibris.com
33131

CONTENTS

Dedication:

To my parents, who led me to believe that my only limitations were those that were self-imposed. (Little did they realize how literally I would take that).

To my respected TCM teachers: Dr. Robert Johns and Pamela Olton, L.Ac.

To Dr. Jerry Alan Johnson, *laoshi* and friend. I thank you for your trust, encouragement, and confidence. Your first direct words to me were, "Don't worry, you have wings," and over the years you taught me how to use them well.

This book is dedicated to Rebecca Blumen. Thank you for absolutely everything and everything absolutely.

FOREWORD

In ancient China, it was customary for a teacher of energetic medicine to pass on the esoteric knowledge and skills of Chinese metaphysical healing to only one gifted student. This "chosen one," had to first prove him or herself worthy of receiving the power and responsibility of this esoteric information. Therefore, the student's integrity, morals, virtue, and skill levels were constantly challenged and tested.

Sometimes it would take a lifetime before the master could find such a student. As a senior instructor and grandmaster of ancient Chinese metaphysical healing, I have been fortunate to have taught and mentored a few talented healers, one of them being Dr. Suzanne Friedman.

When Suzanne first began her training, her dedication and passion for learning ancient Chinese energetic medicine motivated her to study and train extremely hard. With her eyes focused on the goal of mastering energetic diagnostic and treatment modalities, her gifts and comprehension began to rapidly grow. Over the years she has truly blossomed into a powerful healer—one that I am proud of and confident in referring patients to for treatment.

Dr. Suzanne Friedman is one of my most respected graduates, and I can testify to her love, commitment and dedication to her patients' health and well-being. Due to her extensive understanding of traditional Chinese medicine and ancient Chinese energetic medicine, I chose Dr. Friedman to assist me in teaching intensive seminars for several years.

Throughout the following pages, Dr. Friedman meticulously explains to the reader ancient Chinese esoteric medicine theories and exercises. These exercise prescriptions have been effectively used for centuries in clinics and hospitals throughout China for the treatment of disease, and are now substantiated by Western scientific proof gathered through years of clinical research.

Therefore, it is with great pride that I welcome the reader to sit back and enjoy Dr. Friedman's well-researched presentation of Chinese medical qigong exercises, and the theories that substantiate them.

Professor Jerry Alan Johnson, Ph.D., D.T.C.M. (China)
Author of *Chinese Medical Qigong Therapy: A Comprehensive Clinical Text*

INTRODUCTION

The information contained in this book is nothing new. In fact, most of it has been secretly passed down through various daoist lineages over thousands of years. What is new is that modern science now possesses the tools to validate the ancient healing practices contained in this book. This validation has led the National Institutes of Health to dedicate millions of dollars to the research of energy medicine. Qigong doctors and other energy medicine healers welcome this because it means less time spent debating the merits of what we do, and more time spent treating patients.

New patients occasionally ask me for the "proof" behind the qigong exercises I prescribe in my practice. I welcome this inquiry, because knowledge is power, and the more power a patient has, the better the prognosis. Telling someone ⟊ 1 that the exercises are based on thousands of years of clinical research is sometimes not enough. Telling someone that if the exercises did not work they would no longer be passed down or prescribed to hospital patients in China is sometimes ⟊ 2 not enough. Once a patient begins to practice the exercises, that patient will usually feel the proof that he or she is seeking . . . and even that may not be enough. Most of us accept that the body and mind mutually influence and affect each other, but we have a harder time accepting that it is possible to ⟊ 3 *purposefully* harness our mind's power to influence our body, and vice-versa.

For those still questioning, a little story: MDs & Porno

A progressive medical doctor was teaching a continuing education class to her colleagues. She was rattling on about the body-mind connection, and noticed that most of the doctors in the class were either eyeing their watches or falling asleep. The instructor decided that she would have to take a different angle after the lunch break. When they all came back, she took out a pornographic magazine and began reading a graphic story from it. The attendees began squirming in their seats, turning red or white, giggling, and looking around rather perplexedly. The instructor finished the story and asked if anyone felt their temperatures rise. A few people raised their hands. She asked if anyone's heart rate increased. More hands.

She then pointed out that she was able to affect the attendees' bodies with nothing more than sound—sound in the form of the words in the story. By stimulating their minds, the instructor purposefully caused people's bodies to move, their temperatures to rise, their facial color and expression to change, and their heart beat to increase. She noted that if they had read the story without her present, it would have caused the same effects. A simple and sexy illustration of how the mind is linked to the body. They got it.

Another example is the common polygraph test, or lie detector test. Polygraph tests measure physiological responses to questions that elicit emotional reactions. For example, a question that makes a person anxious or nervous will cause a detectable change in heart rate or respiration which is then recorded by the polygraph. The tester asks questions that purposefully manipulate the taker's emotions in order to register a physiological change. The United States court system accepts the results of these tests; tests which confirm that you can alter the body via the mind.

The beauty and advantage of Chinese medicine is its non-linear approach to human physiology. According to Chinese medicine theory, there is no separation between body and mind, and all of the body's internal organs and tissues are either directly or indirectly connected via the body's energetic channels or meridians. This view is confirmed by the living matrix theory of modern physics, which holds that every cell in the body is influenced by and influences every other cell in the body. This theory notes that the liquid crystalline structures of the body, such as cell membranes, connective tissues, microtubules in sensory cells, and DNA, are all capable of sustaining quantum coherence, which accounts for a rapid communication system that exists beyond the nervous system and all well-known communication systems in the body. In other words, the body's tissues have a connection which allows for instantaneous energetic messaging throughout the entire being.

In Chinese medicine and medical qigong theory each yin (solid) internal organ is influenced by, and is considered to "store," a specific emotion. Emotions are stored in the tissues as energetic charges. For example, let's look at anger, which is associated with the liver. When you become angry, the energetic charges associated with your anger cause heat to rise in the body. Heat is a form of energy (along with light, sound, vibration, and color). That heat rises and makes the face warm and red. The body begins to sweat and the breath becomes more deliberate. If that anger is suppressed, the heat and the charges associated with the anger remain in the body's tissues. Over time, this heat from the suppressed anger can build up and become toxic, eventually impeding the biochemical functioning of the body and causing illness.

As taught in basic chemistry, almost every cellular interaction involves the use or the release of energy. Medical qigong consists of specific techniques that use the knowledge of the body's energy fields to purge, tonify (strengthen), and balance these energies. This therapeutic approach addresses the patient's emotional, physical and spiritual imbalances. Positive clinical results are achieved by the recognition and treatment of the person as being more than just the sum of his or her parts.

The exercises in this book utilize breathing techniques, movement, creative visualization and spiritual intent to improve health and control over one's life. Medical qigong movements generate heat and soften the body's connective tissues, which encourages the flushing of intercellular fluid and lymph throughout the body. Qigong movements increase oxygenation of the blood and improve circulation, thereby enhancing lymphocyte production and strengthening the body's immune system. Metabolism is improved, as is the production of cellular energy.

While one can certainly practice qigong exercises without any knowledge of Chinese medicine theory, the practice is deepened tremendously by an understanding of the rationales upon which the exercises are based. When a patient understands how and why a particular exercise works, the therapeutic effect is enhanced because the patient's mind is now focused along with the body's movements. As the Chinese say, "where the mind goes, the qi follows."

What is Medical Qigong?

Medical qigong is one of the four main branches of Chinese medicine, along with acupuncture, herbal therapy and medical massage (*tui na*). It is the energetic foundation from which the other three branches originated. *Qi* means "life-force energy" and *gong* means "skill." Qigong is therefore the skillful practice of gathering, circulating and applying life-force energy. Qigong developed into a systematic healing art for health preservation during the Warring States period in China (476-221 B.C.E.).

There are three main schools of qigong. Martial qigong is the cultivation and storage of energy for use during fighting. Martial qigong consists of dynamic exercises designed to rapidly increase the strength and power for martial arts performance techniques. Spiritual qigong is the cultivation of energy to develop one's connection to one's higher self or higher power. The focus is on *shengong*, the development of "spirit skill" for transformation and enlightenment. This style of qigong involves meditation, breath work, and creative visualization techniques to achieve a state of quiescence. By entering into quiescence, the spirit opens to the voices of the universe.

Medical qigong is the cultivation of energy specifically for health promotion and preservation. It consists of techniques that purge, tonify (strengthen), and balance the body's internal and external energy fields. Medical qigong is a form of self-therapy that combines breathing techniques with movement, creative visualization, and spiritual intent to improve health and control over illness.

According to the laws of physics, matter and energy are interchangeable. In fact, matter is just another form of energy. Matter and energy are in a state of

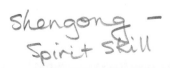
Shengong –
Spirit skill

Vibrational fq = life force energy

Energetic field = biofield = Qi

constant interaction. The flow of qi (energy) produces the magnetic field of the human body, and the magnetic field is a reflection of the energy inherent in the human body. The National Institutes of Health refers to the energetic field produced by the body as a "biofield."   *EMG*

Electrocardiograms (ECG or EKG), electroencephalograms (EEG), and magnetic resonance imaging (MRI) make use of the magnetic and energetic fields of the heart, brain, and body as a whole. Similarly, the earth itself has an electromagnetic field. The atmosphere, also called "the heavens" in early texts, also has its own energetic field. Thousands of years ago, the daoist shamanic doctors devised exercises designed to balance and harmonize human energy with earthly and heavenly energy.

Ancient daoists observed that all matter in the universe was composed of the same substance. To the daoist shamans, the difference between solid, liquid, and gas matter was density and the speed of interaction. Living things all had a particular vibrational frequency, also known as life-force energy, which they called "qi." This vibration, or qi, influences all of the body's energetic and physiological functions. Thus, the daoists would cultivate and regulate the flow of qi to harmonize the body with the emotions, the body with the mind, and ultimately, the body with the spirit.

Medical qigong views each person as possessing three distinct bodies: the material body, or physical body; the energetic body, which controls the material body; and the spiritual body, which controls the energetic body. Qigong exercises address all three bodies in order to rectify imbalance and bring a person closer to physical health and self-actualization.

Medical qigong exercises have been developed and clinically tested over thousands of years. They are prescribed by doctors at medical qigong hospitals in China to treat emotional imbalances and emotionally-induced illnesses. Almost every disease has an emotional component which either led to, or arose from, the illness. When practiced regularly, the exercises lead to a release of stagnant emotions which are causing or can cause depression, anxiety, anger, and physical disease. This release frees up the body's energy for use by the immune system.

There are three objectives for healing disease with medical qigong. First, eliminate internal pathogenic factors (such as the accumulation of excessive emotions), as well as external pathogenic factors from the environment (the invasion of cold, dampness, heat, dryness, for example). Second, increase or decrease a person's qi as needed to counteract the deficient or excess conditions within the body. Third, regulate and balance the patient's yin and yang energy to bring the body back into internal harmony.

Qigong is a means by which anyone can cultivate awareness of the energetic pathways of the body. The goal is to learn how to influence and control the energetic flow within the body to improve immunity, rid the body of illness, and tonify the internal organ systems. Chinese medicine holds that the root cause of disease can be traced to a critical imbalance within the body's vital energies. The practice of medical qigong is one way to prevent or rid the body of disease by establishing a healthy energetic balance between the body's energy fields and the forces of nature and heaven.

The Body as Electromagnetic Matrix

Science as taught in schools is usually divided into three main subjects: biology, chemistry, and physics. Biology emphasizes the physical matrix, consisting of the body's tissues and structures. Chemistry emphasizes the chemical interactions and chemical messengers of the body. It recognizes the ability of the body's cells to communicate within and throughout the entire living system. Students are introduced to the energetic exchanges of ions. An example of which is the transfer of electrons which will either yield more energy or utilize the energy present. These energetic exchanges occur at every moment throughout the body and ensure proper functioning of each cell and organ system.

Physics delves deeper into the 'how' and 'why' of living matter. Recent developments present exciting new views of the universe. What was once thought of as impossible, such as the ability of light to exist as both a particle and a wave, is now considered fact. Moreover, advances in quantum physics, and concepts such as "action at a distance" and "non-locality" confirm the healing principles of certain types of energy work. Medical qigong therapy is one such modality. Research in physics has demonstrated that the presence or absence of the experimenter influences the results of the experiment. Simply put, everything is connected; both within the body and without, near or far.

Basic laws of biomagnetism confirm the role energetics plays in the functioning of the body as a whole. For example, Ampere's Law holds that electrical currents, such as those produced within the body by the activities of the heart, brain, muscles, and other organs, must produce magnetic fields in the space around the body.

Faraday's Law of Induction holds that moving or time-varying magnetic fields in the space around the body must induce current flows within the tissues. This accounts for the effectiveness of magnet therapy. Medical qigong therapy also involves the movement of the doctor's field through that of the patient's, thus inducing current flows throughout the patient's tissues.

Scientists traditionally viewed the nervous and circulatory systems as the primary communication pathways of the body. They have extensively studied the known chemical messengers such as hormones, neurotransmitters, and growth factors. Bioelectrical communication has also been well-documented beyond the nervous system, in which case the water within the body acts as a condenser of energy and a conduit of energy from one place to another.

Energy medicine is now a regular modality utilized in Western hospitals. Electrocardiograms, (ECG or EKG), measure the electrical field and current of the heart that flows throughout the body. Electroencephalograms, (EEG), measure the electric fields put out by the brain and can be registered throughout the body as well. Magnetic Resonance Imaging, (MRI), makes use of the magnetic and energetic fields of the body as a whole. Orthopedic surgeons prescribe the application of "PEMF's" (pulsating electromagnetic fields) to stimulate the repair of fracture non-unions.

One interesting concept shared by both Western science and Chinese medicine is the connection of the heart to the emotions. Scientists have recently demonstrated that there is a relationship between a person's emotional state and the frequency spectrum of the heart. Different emotions affect the signals produced by the heart, and these signals are conducted to every cell in the body and fill the field around the body. Researchers have discovered that some of the heart's neural structures have direct connections with the emotional-cognitive part of the brain called the limbic system. Thus, there is an ongoing dialogue between the heart and brain through these ganglionic connections, and this concept is now called "the functional heart brain." This is but one example of Western research proving the interconnection of the body's tissues and the mind's emotions.

Similarly, in Chinese medicine we say "the heart houses the mind." The word "mind" here means the spirit, not just the brain. In fact, the Chinese word *shen* is associated with both the heart and mind. When one's mind or spirit is agitated, it has a direct effect on the heart. Likewise, when the heart is agitated, it disturbs the spirit and can lead to insomnia, or on the extreme side of the spectrum, insanity. This ancient Chinese concept of the heart and mind (or spirit) connection is thousands of years old, and is exciting to see that Western scientists have found their own way of confirming it.

As modern technology has developed, we are now able to measure the energy fields within and around living systems. This has led to the beginning of a paradigm shift, which is a shift away from merely viewing humans as biochemical beings, and instead seeing humans as energetic beings with high-speed communication pathways and systems that rely on complex energetic exchanges throughout the body. Biochemists have confirmed that all chemical interactions in the body depend on energetic interactions on the molecular level.

Scientists are now extensively studying other forms of energetic signaling beyond the nervous system, such as light, sound, heat, and magnetism. For many centuries, all of these forms of energy have been used in medical qigong therapy for healing purposes. The exercises in this book make use of the clinically confirmed therapeutic effects that these forms of energy have on the body.

Psychosomatics and the Bodymind Concept

Chinese medicine has recognized the body-mind connection for over two thousand years. Ancient Chinese medicine theory sees a person as three inseparable parts: physical, energetic (which includes the emotions), and spiritual. Western medicine has always acknowledged the physical aspect of illness, but can no longer ignore the fact that the body and mind are inextricably linked, and that each influences the other's well-being.

Controlled experiments carried out by allopathic doctors and physicists now confirm the body-mind connection, and the Western medical community is finally acknowledging that emotions can affect one's health. For example, studies have demonstrated that anger can lead to (and meditation can reduce the risk of) heart attacks, that exercise is an anti-depressant, and that laughter boosts the immune system. "Health psychology," "psychoneuroimmunology," and "psychobiology" are three fields of Western medicine which are dedicated to the study of the body-mind connection.

A psychosomatic disorder is defined as a disorder in which the predominant etiological factor in the disease was psychological in origin. Doctors are now starting to accept the logical conclusion gleaned from this concept, which is that physical illness can have psychological roots.

For example, one recent study from the University of Wisconsin-Madison concluded that emotions play an important role in modulating bodily systems that influence our health. Scientists were already aware that pessimists, people rated as sensitive to negative events, show more activity in the right pre-frontal cortex area of the brain. The researchers found that in the six months after volunteers were given a flu shot to elicit an immune response, those who had shown the most powerful right pre-frontal cortex activity also had the worst immune reactions. The reverse was also true for those with the most powerful reactions in their left pre-frontal cortex, the side associated with happy reactions.

While allopathic doctors have made great strides in the treatment of various diseases, incidents of chronic illnesses such as lupus, chronic fatigue syndrome, and fibromyalgia have all been on the rise. Moreover, millions of people are now on prescription drugs, anti-depressants and anti-anxiety medications.

Modern-day stress is taking its toll on our emotional, spiritual and physical bodies. And while medicines may help, they do not necessarily treat the root of the problem, or *why* a person is experiencing certain feelings. My acupuncture mentor, Dr. Robert Johns, used to say that anti-depressants do not make people feel better, they just make people feel less. That is not to say that I oppose the use of these drugs; they have their place and have saved many people from utter despair. I am simply advocating a deeper, more natural way to heal the body's emotional wounds when possible.

Western anatomy demonstrates a connection between the central nervous system (brain and spinal chord) and peripheral nervous system (sympathetic and parasympathetic) and the body's internal organs. The sympathetic nervous system innervates the thymus, bone marrow, spleen and lymph nodes, all of which play a role in the body's immunity. The immune system can both detect and respond to a stress response in the body, as the sympathetic nerves have a direct pathway to lymphocytes (immune cells). The brain itself can control the immune response, as evidenced by studies where electrical stimulation of the hypothalamus resulted in profound changes in immune function. This may be why depression leads to a depressed immune system.

Moreover, stress causes a release of hormones from the adrenal glands. When this happens, the immune system must help rid the body of these hormones, thus diverting it away from its main task of defending the body. This is one of the more obvious connections between stress and immunity. Stress therefore has a measurable, chemical effect on the body which results in stress on the immune system.

Modern physics confirms the teachings of the ancient daoists; that all living matter vibrates at particular wavelengths. Sound vibrates. Color vibrates. Our bodies' cells all vibrate. Modern electrical devices that emit sound are commonly used for this very purpose.

For example, sound vibration is used by Western doctors to shatter gallstones and kidney stones in a procedure known as "lithotripsy." Consumers can purchase electric sonic toothbrushes, which use sound vibration to eradicate plaque from the teeth and below the gum line. In fact, the FDA recently approved a device to treat chronic tennis elbow that uses ultrasonic waves to regenerate healthy tissue to replace inflamed or scarred tendons.

Medical qigong therapy uses sound to purge excess, clear heat, and break apart stagnation. Ancient qigong exercises, known as the "healing sounds," work along these well-recognized scientific principles to release suppressed emotions and blocked energy. That is, vibrations created by sound break apart accumulations and stagnation. Voicing a particular sound adds vibration to a targeted organ system in the body, and breaks apart stagnation, such as heat and anger accumulation in that organ, for example.

The field of psychosomatics is based on the concept that personality and reactions to stress can affect health both for better and for worse. From the 1940's through the 1960's, Franz Alexander and other researchers attempted to test the hypothesis that the cause for seven diseases (asthma, hypertension, rheumatic arthritis, duodenal ulcer, neurodermatitis, thyrotoxicosis and ulcerative colitis) was a specific, intra-psychic conflict derived from early childhood. Alexander acknowledged that disease would only result if there were both a constitutional weakness in the organ system pertaining to that illness and some precipitating circumstance in adult life that reactivated the childhood conflict. Alexander and his colleagues did in fact find similar pathogenic childhood histories along with the repression of certain feelings within each disease category.

In the 1950's Ray Rosenman and Meyer Friedman introduced the term "Type A behavior pattern" to refer to a person with hostile, aggressive, impatient and competitive traits. Men identified as Type A were twice as likely to develop heart disease and five times more likely to have a second myocardial infarction than non-Type A men.

On the other side of the coin, numerous studies, such as those carried out by Dr. Dean Ornish in California, have demonstrated that lifestyle changes such as diet, exercise, meditation and visualization, can reverse heart disease. Reversing heart disease was previously seen as impossible.

When patients feel better or more assured about their treatments, they tend to feel better physically, and have higher rates of healing. Psychologist Leonard Derogatis, in a study of 35 women with metastatic breast cancer, found that the long-term survivors had poor relationships with their physicians, as judged by the physicians. These survivors had asked a lot of questions and expressed their emotions freely. These were women who decided to take control of their healing process, and survived longer as a result.

National Cancer Institute psychologist Sandra Levy has demonstrated that seriously ill breast cancer patients who *expressed* high levels of depression, anxiety, and hostility survived longer than those who showed little distress. This supports medical qigong theories regarding the connection between the release of emotions with an increase in healing.

The studies demonstrating that emotions can lead to illness, and the studies demonstrating that stress-reduction techniques can reverse illness, both validate medical qigong therapy as an effective and powerful treatment modality. This is due to the fact that medical qigong therapy operates on the theory that a large percentage of disease has emotional roots and/or effects, and that healing occurs when repressed emotions are purged from the body.

Groundbreaking Western medical research is now bridging the gap between the theories underlying medical qigong therapy and those of standard, conventional medicine. These findings should serve to strengthen the ties between East and West, and will hopefully result in better and more successful treatment of all disease.

I predict that as Western medicine evolves, and more scientific research is released that confirms the body-mind connection, mainstream acceptance of energy medicine modalities such as medical qigong therapy will only increase.

PART I:

THEORETICAL FOUNDATION

MEDICAL QIGONG THERAPY: MODERN SCIENCE MEETS ANCIENT CHINESE MEDICINE

Improper food and unresolved emotional issues will result in qi blockage and then the portals will be blocked. Cumulative results of constant worry will end in a dormant node developing, hard like a turtle shell but with no pain or itching . . . If at the initial stage of its generation, one eliminates the root of the disease by keeping the heart tranquil and the spirit calm and administers certain treatment, recovery is possible.

Zhu Dan Xi (1281-1358 A.D.), in
The Heart and Essence of Dan Xi's Methods of Treatment

Chairman Mao Tse Tung created what is now called "Traditional Chinese Medicine" out of the many different forms and styles of Chinese medicine that had been practiced throughout China for thousands of years. Mao sought to standardize Chinese medicine so that it could be taught quickly, cheaply, and *en masse.* In doing so, Mao excluded from texts and teachings the ancient parts of Chinese medicine that acknowledge the power of the spirit. He removed many daoist concepts of spirituality, as well as references to theories that could be interpreted as "religious." In a way, Mao took something round, and cut off essential parts of the circle to make it fit into a square. While much traditional medical knowledge was lost or destroyed during the Cultural Revolution, luckily, much also survived.

Medical qigong therapy puts back into Chinese medicine that which was removed when "Traditional Chinese Medicine" was created. It does so by addressing the patient's physical, emotional, and spiritual imbalances according to the daoist shamanic healing concepts that underlie the medicine.

Qigong exercises purge, tonify, or regulate energy within the body. For each exercise, thought (intention), posture, and breath are all crucial. These are known as the "three daoyin."

"Thought" means the active use of imagination, visualization and affirmation. All three change the creative subconscious mind, which in turn re-programs the body. Intent leads the mind (thought), and the mind leads the qi (energy) . We use imagination and visualization to help focus the mind to guide the flow of qi through intended pathways, and to enhance the benefits of the exercise. Affirmation is used as a tool to open the mind to possibilities to which it was closed due to years of conditioning. It is one way to alter one's inner voice towards a new or more positive message.

The Chinese say "When you root the mind, the spirit becomes open to 10,000 voices." The "mind" means your analytical, rational mind. By giving the mind a task, you free the body and become able to feel more from the exercises. You also enhance the ability to tap into your spirit, or your true self. Concentration and thought are both catalysts for chemical reactions in the body. Concentration causes energy to congeal and solidify.

"Posture" means correct physical position. Tension in any area of the body restricts the whole structural system, as the body seeks to balance its structure naturally by shifting its energy and weight. Muscles function to guide the flow of energy through the channels.

Improper posture prevents the flow of energy to a particular area of the body. Proper posture allows energy to flow freely from head to toe, and front to back. In fact, there are eight actions of qi flow: accumulation, dispersion, in-flow, out-flow, rising, sinking, expansion, and contraction.

Form can be thought of as the vessel to which energy can then be added; Dr. Jerry Alan Johnson likens proper form or posture to a well-crafted pitcher which pours freely and does not leak. Proper form allows increased energy cultivation and flow throughout the body.

"Breath" refers to mindful and correct breathing techniques. Qigong masters have always placed a great deal of importance on the breath, believing that a patient's health and emotional condition are deeply affected by breathing patterns and by the amount of oxygen consumed in proportion to the amount of carbon dioxide released. Modern research confirms that relaxed breathing patterns cause every cell to decrease consumption of energy while increasing the storage of energy. Inhalation gathers universal and environmental qi into the body. Exhalation eliminates turbid or toxic qi from the body. In other words, inhalation tonifies and exhalation purges. An even number of each regulates.

While there are many different methods of breath regulation, the method pertinent to most qigong exercises is called "natural abdominal breathing method." The mouth should remain closed, with the tongue placed gently at the junction of the upper palate and the back of the upper teeth. On the inhale, the abdomen fills and expands. On the exhale, the abdomen contracts. The chest barely moves. This will increase the peristaltic action of the digestive system, massage the internal organs, and invigorate and increase the flow of qi from the kidneys into the lower dantian. Babies breathe in this manner. This is also called "diaphragmatic breathing."

Adults, especially those with hypertension, tend to inhale into the chest and shoulders rather than the abdomen. If a patient finds this method difficult, she can practice by lying on her back with a heavy book on the abdomen. When inhaling, the patient tries to raise the book with the expansion of the abdomen. When exhaling, she allows the book to lower as the abdomen relaxes. The chest should neither rise nor fall.

Energetic Anatomy

The Three Dantian

A basic understanding of the body's "energetic pools" enhances qigong practice. As with all martial arts, qigong places great emphasis on the lower dantian. However, many people are unaware of the fact that there are three dantian in the body. "Dantian" literally translates to "elixir field" or "cinnabar field." The three dantian are the body's main energetic reservoirs located in the head, chest, and lower abdomen. They are connected by an energetic pole called the taiji pole which descends from the top of the head to the perineum, through the body's central core. The taiji pole is responsible for absorbing the energy from heaven above and earth below and distributing it into the body's organs and tissues. Qi regulation in and between all three dantian is crucial for mental and physical health.

The upper dantian, also known as "ancestral opening" or "calm fountain," is located in the center of the head, between and behind the eyes. It is considered the door to psychic and intuitive powers, or the ability to "know without knowing." It represents the spiritual aspect of humanity and the connection to the dao, higher power, or infinite void. Excessive concentration and study depletes qi from the upper dantian. Qi is responsible for nourishing the brain and spirit in order to maintain one's mental center. Mental imbalance and depression can result from a lack of qi flow to the upper dantian.

The middle dantian, also known as the "central altar" or "seat of emotion," is located in the center of the chest, between and behind the breasts. This is the chamber of the body's emotional and vibrational power. The middle dantian is where air from the heart and lungs, and food from the digestive system organs are combined and converted into qi energy. Qi disperses from the middle dantian throughout the body. Excess emotions can cause heat or stagnation in the middle dantian, which can impede heart function and digestion.

The lower dantian is also known as the "sea of energy" or "root of life." Generally speaking, it is the area below the navel and above the pubic bone in the lower abdomen. The lower dantian is the root of physical power and the wellspring of human energy. It is the house of kinetic communication and awareness. The goal is to gather qi and store it in the lower dantian for vitality and power. Many people are "in their head" too often, or cannot "turn off" their minds, and sending qi down from the head into the lower dantian helps restore a sense of calm and tranquility. This is known as "rooting" the body's energy.

Meridians: The Body's Energetic Pathways

Meridians are energetic pathways which channel energy throughout the body. Many connect either directly or indirectly with the body's internal organs and the brain. This accounts for communication between different body areas and body organs that would otherwise be considered unconnected. For example, an acupuncturist will place a needle in a patient's foot to alleviate a headache. Needles placed around a patient's right wrist can stop inflammation and pain in the patient's left ankle. Lung problems are often treated along the lung meridian, which means that the doctor will needle a point along the thumb or inner arm.

Some channels are more complex than others. For example, the liver meridian starts from the big toe, ascends the inner leg and wraps around the genitalia. It continues up the torso, alongside the stomach organ, and connects with the liver organ and the gall bladder organ. It then ascends the chest and continues along the posterior aspect of the throat to connect with the eye. From the eye it rises to the top of the head, connects with the Du meridian, and enters the brain. One branch leaves the eye, descends the cheek and curves around the inner surface of the lips. Another ascends the diaphragm and disperses through the lungs. Luckily, it is unnecessary to memorize exact meridian pathways in order to practice qigong. Instead, the practitioner focuses the mind on a generalized pathway such as "up the medial aspect of the leg" or "down from the head to the lower dantian." As stated above, "where the mind goes, the qi follows."

Internal Pathogenic Factors

Traditional Chinese Medicine holds that illness is caused by external pathogenic factors as well as internal pathogenic factors. Internal pathogenic factors can weaken the body's defensive qi which then allows external pathogenic factors to cause physical illness. Other factors (not discussed herein but provided for the sake of completeness) include improper diet, over-exertion, excessive childbearing, traumatic accidents, plague, unbalanced sex life, poison, parasites and iatrogenic disorders.

The six external pathogenic factors arise from climatic changes and are known as: wind, damp, dryness, cold, heat, and summer heat. When the body's defensive qi is deficient, these external pathogenic factors are able to invade the body and cause illness. The weaker the qi, the deeper the pathogenic factor is able to penetrate into the body. In the winter, cold can penetrate the body and cause either a common cold or worsen arthritis. Wind and heat also possess this ability.

The seven internal pathogenic factors arise from excessive internal emotions. They are anger, joy, worry, grief, sadness, fear and shock. If emotions are expressed and released, they do not accumulate and cause mental or physical illness. However, if emotions overwhelm a person, accumulate, or are repressed, they become toxic and affect the corresponding organ or organs of the body.

Accumulation leads to stagnation. A pond becomes stagnant because its water cannot flow or move, as opposed to a river, which is able to maintain clarity through the flow of its water. Likewise, when there is stagnation, the movement of energy is confined. This also confines the space within which the body's cells vibrate. The cells thus begin to vibrate against each other, resulting in the build-up of heat. This heat can then become pathological, surfacing as either physical or psychological illness. High blood pressure and a proclivity towards anger are two manifestations of chronic pathological heat.

Any emotional imbalance can deplete qi or impede the flow of qi in the body. Either creates a functional disorder of the cerebral cortex. Thus, emotional energy can deplete the physical body, which in turn will affect a person's mental and spiritual well-being.

ENERGETIC PSYCHOPHYSIOLOGY

Liu Wan Su (1120-1200 A.D.), in *Za Bin Zhi Li: Illustrations on the Treatment of Miscellaneous Diseases* wrote:

> In relation to the various qi disorders, anger makes the qi ascend, fright makes it chaotic, apprehension makes it descend, taxation makes it issipate, sorrow makes it disperse, joy makes it slack, and thought makes it bind.

The following sections discuss the connection between the body's internal organs and the emotions. An understanding of this connection will aid the practitioner in choosing the exercises most appropriate for his or her condition.

The Liver

The emotion related to the liver is *nu*, which is translated as anger or irritation. Anger makes the qi rise, which accounts for a red face and red eyes. The heat from anger can damage the liver, blood and bile. Anger can invade the digestive organs and cause loss of appetite, diarrhea or constipation.

When the liver is in balance, a person is unselfish, kind, and merciful. When out of balance, a person is stubborn and rude. As the liver rules the blood, stagnation of the flow of liver qi can cause dysmenorrhea (menstrual cramping and pain), and irregular menstruation. Anger causes energy to swell like a wave, rising up the back and over the head.

The Lungs

The emotion related to the lungs is *you* (pronounced "yo"), which is translated as sadness or grief. Pessimism and anxiety are also associated with the lungs. Crying is a reaction to sadness which involves lung energy; just notice a person's chest inflate and deflate as a person cries.

When the lungs are in balance, a person is generous, bright and just. When out of balance, a person is cunning and jealous. Excessive sadness affects the liver as well as the lungs. Sadness as well as anger prevents the smooth flow of liver qi. This causes the qi to stagnate, and depression results. Excess grief from the lungs can also injure the spleen (digestion), causing anorexia and pallor.

Anxiety also blocks lung qi and suppresses respiration. It weakens the body's defensive qi. Anxiety also affects the large intestine, leading to constipation, irritable bowel, Crohn's disease, and other bowel diseases.

Grief obstructs the flow energy. It has a thick, heavy, gelatinous quality, and moves things downward. A person feels heavy, and the head hangs down. Eyes too look downwards.

The Kidneys

The emotion related to the kidneys is *kong*, which is translated as fear. Paranoia is also related to the kidneys. When the kidneys are in balance, a person is peaceful, soft and tender. When out of balance, a person is ignorant, troublesome and arrogant.

Fear can cause incontinence (loss of bladder or bowel control), knee weakness, and renal failure. When fear injures the liver, it causes spasms and irregular menstruation. Fear can invade the gallbladder, making it difficult to make decisions. When fear affects the heart, it will disturb the spirit and speech, and is reflected in the eyes.

The energetic pattern of fear is cold, and inward moving. It travels from the eyes down the front of the body, through the heart, and into the groin. Fear should be distinguished from sudden fright, or intense shock. Sudden fright or shock affects the heart and then the kidneys. The energy seizes the center, startles the spirit, scatters qi and injures the heart. If the shock continues, it will mutate into chronic fear and damage kidney qi.

The Spleen

The emotion related to the spleen is *si*, which is translated as worry, pensiveness, contemplation and over-thinking. When the spleen is in balance, a person is forgiving, sincere and willing to compromise. When out of balance, a person is suspicious and self-centered.

Worry prevents qi flow and can lead to in stomach disorders such as indigestion, ulcers, poor appetite, constipation and diarrhea. The energetic pattern of worry causes energy rising from the earth to stagnate in the middle dantian, which weakens the body's defensive qi.

The Heart

The emotion related to the heart is *xi,* which is translated as joy or excitement. When the heart is in balance, a person is open-minded, peaceful and trustful. When out of balance, a person is confused, doubtful and greedy.

Excess joy, laughter, and over-excitement can injure the heart, causing it to beat erratically. Likewise, anxiety surrounds and agitates the heart, interfering with heart qi. The energy of joy (when in balance) ripples out from the body's center in all directions. It is a light-natured energy that causes qi to move more slowly. It touches others and is reflected back to the person expressing the emotion.

Energetic Psychology

As previously mentioned, the five emotions are anger, joy, fear, worry and grief. Before a person acquires or experiences these five emotions, a person's heart is first and foremost affected. When the heart is affected, it sets an emotional cycle into play.

There are three emotions the heart will experience when a person first feels hurt. They are abandonment, betrayal and/or rejection. After this immediate reaction comes anger, followed by grief and despair, and then possibly fear. Anger involves the liver. Grief involves the lungs. Fear involves the kidneys.

The heart stores long-term memories, and the kidneys store short-term memories. Emotions and the memories attached to them will pool to the area located below the heart, called the "yellow court." It is called the yellow court because in ancient times the heart was also known as "suspended gold." This is the area where memories are stored when a person is not ready to deal with them. The yellow court is a temporary holding zone for the emotions, and it is the physiological location of repressed memories.

The Ethereal and Corporeal Souls: Hun and Po

We are very much familiar with the scenario of a little angel sitting on one shoulder, and a little devil sitting on the other shoulder. The little angel tells the person to do what is right; the devil tells the person to do what is best for one's self. Similarly, Chinese medicine has ancient energetic concepts that reflect the inner angel/devil dichotomy, however neither is considered evil.

The po, also known as the corporeal soul, is a person's animal nature. The po is the inner, instinctive protector. It is what is responsible for actions taken to defend one's self; it is sometimes called the angry general. The po is similar to the little devil, with the judgment of good and evil removed. The po does not counsel you to do evil, but it is your instinct to do what is necessary to protect yourself. The po also registers psychological pain.

The hun, also known as the ethereal soul, is a person's energetic inner guide; one's minister of wisdom. It controls sleep and dreaming and registers physical pain. The hun are located in each of the three dantian, and are associated with, or "housed by" the liver.

The hun in the upper dantian connects with the dao, a higher power, or the infinite void. It is a component of your intuitive self. The hun in the middle dantian is connected with the desire for order, compassion and integrity. It is a component of your empathetic self. The hun in the lower dantian is connected with the enjoyment of life. It is a component of your kinesthetic self.

For balance, a person must make the po listen to the hun. For example, when a person gets drunk, the hun is said to leave the body, and the po takes over. Frequently, drunken behavior is evidence that the hun has left and the po is in charge.

One way to calm the po is through conscious breathing techniques. This is because the po is associated with, or "housed by" the lungs. When a patient feels himself getting angry and his defense mechanisms begin to impede a balanced reaction, slow, deep breathing, coupled with sending the rising hot energy down from the head, will help him stay in control and "keep his cool." In other words, this technique will tame the po.

PART II:

GETTING STARTED—MEDICAL QIGONG
SELF-REGULATION THERAPY:
QIGONG EXERCISE PRESCRIPTION
THEORY & GUIDELINES

The *Dao Yin Tu,* from the second century, B.C.E., illustrates over 45 qigong postures and the diseases they treat. Over half of the illustrated postures are animal movements. Movement stimulates and increases the flow of the body's qi and blood. In the classic text, *Spring and Autumn Annals*, it is written that "flowing water never stagnates, and the hinges of an active door never rust."

Although acupuncture and herbs can also move qi and blood, they fail to address a patient's lifestyle and emotional or stress patterns, which are often major contributing factors to illness. Medical qigong doctors prescribe physical therapy, exercise, and meditations as part of the overall treatment strategy to counter a sedentary, stressed, or unhealthy lifestyle.

The three main rules for treatment with medical qigong exercise prescriptions are:

1. Tonify the deficient organs and organ systems with color visualization by using the mind's intention to focus on moving qi to the area, thus strengthening and illuminating deficient tissues.
2. Purge the excess organs and organ systems with sound resonation by using the mind's intention to focus on moving qi out from an excess organ by resonating and draining the area.
3. Regulate the body's yin and yang organs with qigong by using the mind's intention to balance the energetic fields by moving the qi up and down, right and left, and inside and outside the tissues.

Medical qigong exercise prescriptions are designed to disperse qi and blood stagnation, to tonify the internal organs and organ systems, and to enhance the functioning of the autonomic nervous system. By stimulating the patient's body, the exercises will eliminate fatigue as normal body function is restored. Another important therapeutic effect is immune enhancement by increasing cellular energy and circulating lymph.

There are five stages of healing awareness in medical qigong self-regulation therapy. These are transitions achieved through practice.

1. The patient is taught to increase his or her awareness of the body and its current condition.
2. The patient is taught to cleanse and purify the body's energetic fields, ridding the body of qi stagnation and toxic pathogenic factors.
3. The patient is taught to strengthen and recharge his or her body to replenish the qi.
4. The patient is taught to circulate the qi internally and externally, moving any stagnant qi and strengthening the body.
5. The patient is taught to dissipate any excess qi from the body with self-massage.

The exercise prescriptions in this book enable a patient to reinforce treatments performed by a qigong doctor, acupuncturist, or other health provider, and prevent the patient's energy from reverting back to old, destructive patterns. The qigong doctor selects the proper exercise prescription(s) to fit the patient's illness. The patient is dissuaded from practicing at random, in order to avoid pathological changes or qi deviations which can arise from improper practice.

Given the paucity of qigong doctors in the United States, this book is designed to ensure that practitioners and patients are led to appropriate exercises that would normally be prescribed after a qigong treatment.

POSTURAL DAOYIN TRAINING

The goal of postural daoyin training is to promote qi circulation and regulation. It involves learning techniques to guide qi through movement and changes in the electromagnetic fields of the hands and body. Proper posture and alignment are imperative and ensure the efficacy of the exercises.

Correct posture regulates the heart and calms the mind. This makes it easier to lead the flow of qi downward and aids smooth qi and blood circulation. There is a proper sequence of relaxation for energy circulation. The muscles are relaxed, followed by the tendons and ligaments, then the nerves, and finally the bones.

When the qi and blood flow through the channels, the practitioner may experience bodily sensations such as heat, tingling, vibration, or fullness. When qi flows through the nerves, the practitioner may experience an energetic current or electric surge through the body or extremities.

Static postural daoyin training involves the cultivation of a quiescent state while lying down, sitting, or standing. It is used to build and strengthen the practitioner's internal qi in the lower dantian for circulation throughout the body. Meditation and visualization exercises fall under this category.

While static qigong exercises accumulate and strengthen internal qi, dynamic postural daoyin training involves the channels, collaterals, muscles and bones. The more dynamic the movements, the more the qi will be transformed inside the body. The exercises affect muscular tension, weight distribution, and the function of the internal organs. Dynamic qigong exercises increase the circulation of qi and blood in the channels and throughout the body.

There are three main components of postural daoyin training. They are as follows:

1. Proper beginning posture. Proper posture will help the practitioner to relax the mind and release tension from the body, as well as focus on a specific goal for training.
2. Proper breathing method. When the qi flows freely, the practitioner focuses on each inhalation and exhalation with the goal of tonification, purgation, or regulation of qi.
3. Proper closing posture. To root the body's energy in the lower dantian for storage. This avoids the creation of an excess condition or qi deviations from the gathered qi.

A fourth component must always be considered in addition to the above three. That component is intention, or focus of mind. The exercises cannot be considered qigong without the force of the mind to guide the qi. The enhancement of qi flow via visualization and intention cannot be overemphasized.

The practitioner will choose the proper posture and duration of practice based on his or her own particular strength and condition. For example, weaker patients will be taught exercises that can be performed lying down. Sitting is encouraged for those who feel able. Standing is the most favorable posture, but only if the body's condition allows. For weaker patients, and for static qigong in general, the emphasis is on visualization and qi flow rather than physical movement. For stronger patients, the emphasis is on visualization, qi flow and physical movement.

Sitting is the most commonly used position for medical qigong meditation. This position helps the patients to relax and focus the mind. A patient can sit on a cushion or chair, but should try to have the buttocks slightly higher than the knees. This will form a triangle between the knees and the lower dantian, which establishes a firmer connection to the earth energy. This also allows the qi from the earth to flow freely from the knees and coccyx into the body. In addition, if the feet are firmly planted on the ground, it will enhance the qi flow from the earth into the body.

Standing exercises (both dynamic and static) are the most tonifying in terms of gathering qi. Standing allows the regulation and promotion of qi flow. Proper standing posture, with the body relaxed and bones stacked on top of each other from the ground up, helps normalize blood pressure and calm the mind. The body should be relaxed and rooted into the ground like a tree with roots shooting deep into the earth.

When beginning standing meditation or dynamic exercises, patients should first relax, sink, and shift their body weight back and forth between the balls of their feet and their heels. This practice provides a subtle massage of the internal organs and helps dispel energetic blockages. Shifting forward causes the energy from the front of the body to flow downwards and sink, and shifting backwards causes the energy from the back of the body to flow downwards and sink. This practice is enhanced by inhaling when shifting backwards and exhaling when shifting forwards. The qi should flow back and forth like gentle waves in the ocean.

Women who are menstruating should practice qigong exercises and meditation while standing rather than sitting to avoid blocking energy circulation in the lower abdomen. In addition, at the end of an exercise program, women who are menstruating should store the energy in their middle dantian rather than their lower dantian.

ESSENTIAL GUIDELINES FOR SELECTING THE PROPER EXERCISES IN THIS BOOK

When prescribing medical qigong exercises, it is important to have a clear understanding of the patient's constitution and physical or psychological abilities. Proper diagnosis is essential for proper treatment. For example, an asthma attack can be categorized as an excess condition, but it may be due to an underlying lung and kidney deficiency. Therefore, one must determine whether the body is strong enough to focus on purging the excess, whether the focus should be on tonifying the deficiency, or whether both must be carried out in a particular sequence. If you are unsure whether you have an excess or deficient condition, please seek out the advice of a licensed acupuncturist or medical qigong doctor.

Every qigong regimen should begin with a basic purging exercise. Purging exercises cleanse the body of pathogenic qi and calm and ready the mind. There is a Chinese saying: "Do not put clean water in a dirty glass." In other words, before you attempt to gather qi, you must cleanse the vessel in which it will be stored. The opening exercise called Pulling Down Heavens is sufficient for this purpose. You may choose the appropriate purging exercises for the condition to be addressed after completing Pulling Down Heavens.

After purgation, the body-mind-spirit is prepared for tonification, or strengthening, exercises. The goal is to strengthen and stabilize the internal organ systems and qi and blood flow throughout the body. As indicated above, it must first be determined that tonification exercises are warranted.

Regulation exercises neither tonify nor purge, but rather balance yin and yang energy. The regulation may lead to the strengthening of weakness and the sedation of excess, and therefore these exercises are particularly safe when there is doubt about whether a condition is an excess or deficiency condition. Regulation exercises follow tonification and purgation exercises, with the goal of re-establishing internal balance and homeostasis by circulating energy through the body. The patient should conclude with an appropriate closing posture to end and seal the practice. Pulling Down Heavens is an exemplary closing exercise.

Patients with serious, life-threatening illnesses, such as cancer, should not practice general qigong exercise protocols. They should immediately discontinue their regular qigong routines, and practice only exercises and meditations specifically designed for cancer or for their particular disease.

A basic Chinese medicine concept is that if a patient has an excess condition (such as cancer), a doctor must be careful not to tonify that condition. Tonifying exercises practiced in a haphazard manner can possibly result in unintentionally growing or strengthening an excess disease, for example. Likewise, if a patient has a deficient condition, emphasis on purgation is inappropriate, as purging exercises may drain much needed energy from an already weakened body. Exercises for cancer and other serious illnesses are beyond the scope of this book. Therefore, I must strongly discourage these patients in particular from randomly choosing the exercises contained herein.

UNIVERSAL QIGONG PRACTICE KEYS

The following is a list of practice keys designed to function as a quick reference tool. It contains essential guidelines to help ensure that the selected exercises are appropriate and are not contraindicated for the patient's condition. Please familiarize yourself with these concepts before designing an exercise self-treatment plan or a treatment plan for patients.

- Sound purges, and color tonifies. Therefore, use sound to purge excess and color to strengthen deficiency. Selection of the proper sound or color is based on the organ or organ systems involved according to five element theory. When unsure of which color to use, choose white.

- If there is qi or energy deficiency, the focus should be on tonification exercises and meditations.
- If there is an excess of emotions, such as worry, anxiety, or anger, purgation exercises should be emphasized.
- Unless otherwise indicated, practice abdominal breathing throughout the regimen. (The abdomen is pushed out on the inhale, and pulled in on the exhale).
- Where there is prolapse, or sinking, choose exercises that raise qi. Where there is abnormal rising (also known as rebellious qi), such as high blood pressure with a red face, anger outbursts, coughing, nausea or vomiting, choose exercises that ground and root qi.
- For heat conditions, choose cooling colors for qigong meditation practice, such as blue, rather than warming colors, such as red. If it is an excess heat condition, then purgation is appropriate. If the heat is caused by deficient yin (not enough moisture to maintain temperature balance), meditations and exercises which tonify yin are appropriate. People with high blood pressure should visualize pink rather than red whenever red is called for in a meditation.
- Excess cold conditions are rare in this modern age of central heating. However, deficient cold conditions, which are constitutional or caused by adrenal burn-out, are not uncommon. Warming colors and tonification of kidneys are appropriate.
- When in doubt, regulation exercises are safest because they have the effect of balancing yin and yang energy.
- Do not practice when exceedingly hungry, emotional, or tired. One's mind should be tranquil, and the body should be able to relax. Wait 30 to 60 minutes after eating to begin your practice.
- Under no circumstances should you practice under the influence of drugs or alcohol.
- Where there's pain, there's no gain. Do not "push through" pain. Qigong practice requires that you listen to what the body is trying to tell you. If you are in pain, stop immediately. Muscle soreness after rigorous exercise is to be expected when first beginning qigong. However, sharp or stabbing pain means that the posture is either incorrect or the exercise is inappropriate for one's physical condition.
- Changes in digestion, sleep patterns, urination, and emotional releases can all result from qigong practice. For example, exercises which purge toxins can cause cloudy urination or diarrhea. However, if you have any questions or concerns whatsoever regarding such changes, you are strongly encouraged to seek the advice of a health professional. Never guess or assume when it comes to your health and well-being.

PART III:

GENERAL EXERCISE PRESCRIPTIONS

The Rules of Proper Medical Qigong Structure: Wuji Posture

The following is a beginner's list for proper standing posture, which is called Wuji posture. Wuji posture is the foundation for all dynamic and quiescent standing exercises. This posture maximizes relaxation and qi flow.

1. Stand with the feet flat
2. Bend the knees
3. Relax the hips
4. Close the anal sphincter
5. Relax the waist
6. Tuck in the chest & relax upper limbs
7. Suspend the head & tuck the chin
8. Close the eyes for inner vision
9. Touch the tongue to the upper palate

Each of these rules is described in detail as follows:

Rule 1 - Stand with the feet flat

Stand with the feet flat parallel to the outside of the shoulders. Weight should be distributed evenly on the centers of both feet and toes should be pointing forwards.

The toes softly grasp the ground to keep the body firmly rooted yet relaxed. Rigid or tense feet disrupt the flow of qi from the earth into the body.

The feet may vibrate or feel hot while training. This is a normal reaction to correct postural training and is beneficial as it dissolves any calcium deposits accumulated in the extremities of the feet.

Rule 2 - Bend the Knees

The knees should be slightly bent and facing the same direction as the feet. Never bend the knees past the toes. Many people develop knee problems from various forms of exercise because they bend their knees too far forward or allow their knees to twist. Relaxing the knee joint increases the qi and blood flow through the legs.

Rule 3 - Relax the Hips

Drop the buttocks slightly while sinking the qi from the upper torso into the lower dantian, and relax the hips. Try to reduce the curve in the lower back while keeping the upper body from bending forward or backward. The buttocks should be gently tucked in to help strengthen the spine and focus the qi in the lower dantian.

You may also imagine a heavy weight hanging from the coccyx (tailbone). As the weight pulls down, tilt the sacrum under the body.

Rule 4 - Close the Anal Sphincter

The anus is known as the lower bridge, as it is where the yang and yin channels meet and combine. Gently closing the anal sphincter seals the gathered qi in the body. Although the anal sphincter is held closed, it is important that the perineum and buttocks remain relaxed. Patients may initially find it difficult to use abdominal breathing while keeping the anus closed. Be assured that it will rapidly become an unconscious reflex after regular practice.

Rule 5 - Relax the Waist

Relaxing the waist sinks the qi into the lower dantian. Relax the waist by relaxing the hips and bending the knees. When the waist is relaxed, the spine will stand straight and upright.

The abdomen is considered to be a furnace for refining qi. The waist area is the residence of the kidneys and mingmen fire (gate of vitality or destiny) and is an important junction for qi and blood circulation.

Rule 6 - Tuck in the Chest & Relax Upper Limbs

The shoulders should be tucked back and then down, without "puffing" out the chest. On the inhale, fill the abdomen with breath while relaxing the chest with minimal movement. The back should be open and relaxed while you sink the shoulders. When the chest and back are without tension, the heart and lungs are able to function more efficiently, and circulation of energy in the Ren and Du channels is improved.

When the neck is loose and the shoulders are in proper posture, qi will flow freely into the arms. The elbows are slightly bent and held at the sides of the body with palms facing the legs or facing backwards.

Rule 7 - Suspend the Head & Tuck the Chin

Visualize the body as if suspended by a string connected to the crown point (Du 20) on the head. The crown point should be directly above the body. This will elongate the spine and tuck the chin. Slightly tucking the chin and stacking the vertebrae on top of one another facilitates qi and blood flow through the spinal column and brain. Feel the spine elongate with each breath. Check each part of the body to ensure that all muscles are relaxed.

Rule 8 - Close the Eyes for Inner Vision

It is easier to feel or guide inner qi circulation with the eyes closed. The eyes therefore remain closed during meditations and visualizations.

When regulating the body's energy, during dynamic exercises for example, the eyes remain soft and slightly open. Light is yang, and dark is yin, and qi is balanced by the combination of both.

Rule 9 - Touch the Tongue to the Upper Palate

When the tongue touches the upper palate behind the teeth, it connects the Ren and Du meridians like a circuit and enhances qi circulation in the front and back of the body. The lips are gently closed and the teeth slightly touch. This seals in the qi and prevents it from leaking, as does closing the anal sphincter.

Opening Exercise: Pulling Down the Heavens

This exercise should be used to begin every qigong practice without exception. It is a purging exercise which cleanses the internal organs, eliminates turbid qi, enhances qi flow downward through all meridians and tissues, and calms the mind. One set consists of focusing the qi down the front, the back, and then center of the body. Pulling Down the Heavens will ground and ready you for the practice, and can be used as a solo exercise as well.

Description:
1. Begin in Wuji posture with eyes slightly open to absorb qi from the environment into the lower dantian. Breathe using abdominal breathing. Inhale and exhale through the nose.

2. Inhale and raise arms out to the sides with palms facing downward. Absorb the energy from the earth into body through the palms. At shoulder height, turn the palms up and absorb qi from the heavens (universal energy) into the body as your hands continue to rise overhead.

3. Exhale and begin descending the palms down the front of the body with right and left hand fingertips pointing at each other. Palms face down and direct the qi flow down the entire front of the body and deep into the earth.

Inhale and begin sequence again. The second time through the energy is directed down the back of the body from the back of the head down into the earth. The third time through, the energy penetrates the crown point (Du 20, the highest point of the head) and passes through the entire inside of the body and deep into the earth. As a stand-alone exercise, practice for 36 sets.

Visualize the gathering of qi on the inhale, and the lowering of qi on the exhale. When sending the energy down the front and back of the body, feel each muscle relaxing as the energy passes it. When pulling energy through the center of the body, imagine it coating, cleansing, and soothing all internal organs. Be sure to visualize the energy sinking deep into the earth with each pass.

To end the exercise, relax whole body and return to Wuji posture. Imagine a thick healing mist within and around the body.

This exercise is sufficient to purge the body before beginning tonification exercises for people who are generally healthy and wish to practice qigong for health maintenance purposes.

For people with specific health conditions, at this point you will turn to the sections of the book which address your condition, and continue according to the instructions contained therein.

GENERAL PURGING EXERCISES

HEALING SOUNDS TO PURGE ORGAN EXCESS AND IMBALANCE

Healing Sound Therapy

From as far back as the Qin Dynasty (221-207 BC), healing sounds have been recorded and used for healing purposes. Sound vocalization has a direct effect on the body's sympathetic and parasympathetic nerves. Emphasis is placed on the connection of mind, breath, and imagination to the area of focus. You must feel enveloped in sound, vibration and energy while intoning the therapeutic sounds. Healing sounds should be practiced before tonification and regulation exercises.

Contraindications for the Healing Sound Therapy:

Do NOT practice sound therapy if any of the following apply:
1. Broken or fractured bones
2. Acute stage of illness
3. Pregnancy
4. Menstruation

Proper Number of Breaths for Healing Sound Practice: Begin with a minimum of 3-6 vocalizations before proceeding on to the next sound. If you are practicing on a daily basis, 24 vocalizations should be the maximum per sound or sounds you choose.

Tones: A rising tone will cause the qi to ascend; a descending tone will cause the qi to descend. When in doubt, use a straight tone.

Breath and Mind Control: While inhaling imagine breathing in white light healing energy through your nose and absorbing this healing qi into the target area, vibrating it. When exhaling sound, imagine breathing out dark turbid qi through the mouth. This visualization is essential.

The Six Healing Sounds
1. **"Xu" (pronounced "shu") Purges the Liver:** The xu sound relieves liver qi stagnation, heat, anger, irritability and impatience, and helps certain visual distortions.

    1. Begin with Pulling Down Heavens
    2. Interlace fingers, raise the hands over the head until elbows are straight, and twist hands so palms face the sky
    3. Lean slightly to the left to open the liver (which is located on the right side)
    4. Inhale qi in the form of white light to the liver organ
    5. Exhale the xu sound while visualizing dark turbid qi and unwanted emotions being released from the liver and exiting the mouth with the breath
    6. Repeat 6 to 24 times
    7. End with Pulling Down Heavens before beginning next sound or exercise

2. **"Ha" Relieves the Heart** The ha sound relieves fire and anxiety from the heart, expels heat from the body, and improves poor circulation.

    1. Begin with Pulling Down Heavens
    2. Raise arms above head with elbows slightly bent

3. Palms face forward and tilt slightly towards the sky
4. Inhale qi in the form of white light to the heart
5. Exhale the ha sound and visualize dark turbid qi, heat, and anxiety exiting via the mouth and palms
6. Repeat 6 to 24 times
7. End with Pulling Down Heavens before beginning next sound or exercise

3. **"Hu" Aids the Spleen:** The hu sound (pronounced "who") improves sluggish digestion, helps reduce heartburn, and relieves dampness, gas and bloating.

1. Begin with Pulling Down Heavens
2. Interlace fingers, raise the hands over the head until elbows are straight, and twist hands so palms face the sky
3. Lean slightly to the right to open the spleen (which is located on the left side)
4. Inhale qi in the form of white light to the area of the spleen, stomach and pancreas
5. Exhale the hu sound while visualizing dark turbid qi being released from the spleen and stomach and exiting the mouth with the breath
6. Repeat 6 to 24 times
7. End with Pulling Down Heavens before beginning next sound or exercise

4. **"Sh" (pronounced "shhh") Drains the Lungs:** The sh sound opens the lungs, relieves phlegm, and dispels grief.

1. Begin with Pulling Down Heavens
2. Raise arms above head with elbows slightly bent
3. Bend elbows until hands are on either side of head, with palms facing forward and tilting slightly towards the sky
4. Inhale qi in the form of white light to the lungs
5. Exhale the sh sound while visualizing turbid qi and grief leaving via the mouth and palms
6. Repeat 6 to 24 times
7. End with Pulling Down Heavens before beginning next sound or exercise

5. **"Chri" (pronounced "chree") Warms the Kidneys:** The chri sound expels chills, and maintains internal heat of the lower dantian and Mingmen

Fire. This should only be practiced with a diagnosis of kidney yang deficiency, excess fear, or excess cold.

1. Begin with Pulling Down Heavens
2. Stand with knees together
3. Place right palm on right knee and left palm on left knee, elbows slightly bent
4. Inhale qi in the form of white light to the kidneys (the mid-to-low back area)
5. Inhale qi in the form of warm white light to the kidneys
6. Exhale the sound chree out of the mouth, and release cold turbid qi and fear from the kidneys
7. Repeat to 24 times
8. End with Pulling Down Heavens before beginning next sound or exercise.

6. **"Xi" (pronounced "she") Cools the Triple Burners:** The xi sound eliminates systemic excess heat, cools rheumatoid arthritis and tuberculosis, and is always prescribed for patients undergoing radiation or chemotherapy, as it disperses the toxic heat from the tissues. This exercise is practiced while lying on your back or while performing Pulling Down Heavens, depending on the patient's constitution. If lying down, follow the instructions regarding breath and visualization. The body does not move if you are lying down.

1. Begin with Pulling Down Heavens
2. Inhale white healing light into entire body as you raise the hands up (the gathering part of Pulling Down Heavens)
3. Exhale the xi sound and visualize heat and turbid qi being released down the entire body and deep into the ground as the hands lower
4. Repeat 6 to 24 times (if undergoing chemotherapy or radiation, 36 times is advisable and can be broken up into three times per day)
5. End with Pulling Down Heavens before beginning next sound or exercise

Once you are sufficiently purged, you may turn to the following qigong exercise sections.

GENERAL TONIFICATION AND REGULATION EXERCISES FOR HEALTH MAINTENANCE

The following exercise, entitled Opening and Closing the Three Burners, is provided as a dynamic qigong tonification exercise. It can be modified depending on the particular illness. For example, if there is an excess disease or imbalance in the upper burner, then the focus is on releasing the excess with the exhale. If there is a deficient disease in the middle burner, then the focus would be on the inhale to gather qi to the area.

The intermediate level of this exercise adds color on the inhale and/or sound on the exhale, depending again on the patient's condition. It is important to become comfortable with the basic exercise before adding to it. If you are ready to add color or sound, please refer to the sections that clarify which sounds and colors are appropriate for specific internal organs. Keep in mind that sound is never used for deficient conditions, and color is never used for purely excess conditions.

Opening and Closing the Three Burners: The three burners are three distinct areas of the body which house the internal organs. The upper burner is the area where the heart and lungs reside. The middle burner is where the digestive organs reside. The lower burner is where the genital organs and lower portion of the large intestine reside. This exercise set regulates the body's yin and yang energy, strengthens the yin organs, harmonizes the yang organs, and opens the Ren and Du meridians. It will regulate the flow of energy in the triple burners (*san jiao*), and the increase in flow will help cool liver heat. There is an ancient saying, "Open, close, and come and go, one hundred illnesses will be healed."

When opening, the qi circulates to the surface. When closing, the qi sinks deeper and gathers into the tissues and organs, and penetrates the bones. This exercise will help hone the focus of intention, and facilitates an increase in the body's wei qi (defensive qi) field to prevent illness.

It is assumed that you are standing in Wuji posture and that you have already completed the Pulling Down Heavens opening exercise for purgation before beginning the exercises in this section.

The Upper Burner

1. Standing in Wuji, raise both arms to shoulder level and vigorously shake hands with palms facing down. Focus on sending energy and awareness to the center of the palms, (where the laogong or Pericardium 8 point is located) for a few minutes. The palms should become warm with qi.
2. Bring both hands close together with palms facing each other in front of the upper part of the sternum (the manubrium). The area is lower than the throat but higher than between the breasts. Fingers face upwards. The eyes gently gaze at the space between the palms, and then close for inner vision.
3. Inhale and focus on the center of palms, and visualize an energetic ball pulsating and growing thicker with qi. Exhale and slowly pull hands and arms apart, imagining the ball of qi stretching and expanding. Visualize the ball growing to penetrate and open the entire chest area. The front

and back of the upper torso expand and release as the hands separate and open. Feel the mind expand. The energy expands out from the body in all directions.

4. Inhale, and slowly bring both palms together, condense and gather the qi, returning it to the energetic ball between your hands. As the hands come together, the mind and body settle and the energy condenses in the upper torso. Focus on the inside of the body, as if you are sealed off from the external world.

When exhaling and separating hands, imagine the qi penetrating the entire body from front to back while releasing toxicity and excess heat. When inhaling, visualize the qi filling and strengthening every cell in the body.

Repeat 18 times before lowering hands to the middle burner.

The Middle Burner
1. Lower the hands to the stomach area (below the sternum) while still holding a small energy ball. The wrists should relax so that the fingers are no longer pointing directly upward but instead rotated very slightly forward. The eyes gently gaze at the space between the palms and then close. Inhale.
2. Exhale and slowly separate the palms. Visualize the energy ball stretching pressing against the palms. Feel the energy blow through the center of the body like wind, purging toxicity and excess heat.
3. Inhale and bring both palms together, condensing the energy ball back between the hands and feeling every cell in the body filled with qi.
   Repeat 18 times before sinking hands to the lower burner.

The Lower Burner
1. Lower the hands to the area in front of the pubic bone. The wrists are relaxed and the fingers are tilted further towards the ground. The eyes gently gaze at the space between the palms and then close. Inhale.
2. Exhale and slowly pull palms apart as the energy expands to fill the void. Feel excess heat and toxic energy being purged from the body.
3. Inhale and bring palms together, re-forming the energetic ball. Feel the qi penetrate deep into the body, nourishing every cell.
   Repeat 18 times. To end the exercise, perform the Pulling Down Heavens exercise to sink the qi for storage in the lower dantian.

Organ Self-Massage
The following exercises are commonly practiced to help increase and target energy for self-healing. Organ self-massage prescriptions can be practiced alone

or within a qigong program, as they purge, tonify, and regulate the five yin organ systems. These exercises are safe to choose where there is a combination of excess and deficiency, or where a practitioner is unsure of the exact nature of a disorder or imbalance. They can be performed lying down, sitting up, or standing. The regulation section of each organ massage brings blood and qi to the targeted area. The point respiration section of each organ massage helps clean and purify the organ of turbid qi accumulation. Practitioners can choose just one set or all of the sets listed below. For clinical therapy, perform the exercise(s) three times a day.

Heart Massage

1. Stand in Wuji posture and begin to breathe deeply. Relax the mind and visualize your body melting into the ground on the exhale.
2. Heart Regulation: Place one palm on top of the other hand and hold both hands over the heart. Massage in 12 circular rotations clockwise to the left, and then 12 times counterclockwise around the heart area. If you are able to sense the qi in the body without touching, the hands do not need to touch the body as they circle. If you are still developing your energetic sensitivity, you can gently touch the skin with the bottom hand as it circles. Regardless of which you choose, focus the mind's intention on the heart, visualizing the energy of the heart circulating and flowing along with the movement of your hands. The rotating action around the heart promotes blood circulation and disperses blood stasis.
3. Point Respiration: The hands remain one on top of the other, held in front of the heart. Concentrate the mind and focus your intention on the heart area and organ. Inhale and exhale through the nose. As you inhale, breathe into the heart organ. Exhale while lightly pressing or squeezing the area of the heart with the hands, imagining healing light radiating out of the heart as you press. Inhale and lift the hands away from the heart as you visualize healing light flowing into the heart like a bellows. Repeat for 12 inhalations and exhalations. Close by leading the qi down into the lower dantian on an exhale.
4. End with Pulling Down the Heavens: When lowering the arms in front of the torso on the exhale, imagine the energy of the heart like water, melting and flowing down with the hands and filling the lower dantian. The qi is stored in the lower dantian so that the gathered energy will not be easily dispersed.

Liver Massage

1. Stand in Wuji posture and begin to breathe deeply. Relax the mind and visualize your body melting into the ground on the exhale.

2. Liver Regulation: Place the right hand on the liver and the left hand on the right hand. (The liver is located on the right side of the body approximately where the ribcage ends). Massage in circular rotations clockwise to the left 12 times. Then massage in counter-clockwise circles 12 times. Keep the mind focused on the liver and try to sense the qi moving in the area of the liver.

3. With your hands over the liver: inhale and imagine healing light filling the liver from the breath and from your hands. Exhale through the mouth, and imagine turbid qi leaving the liver via the exhaled breath. This visualization and breath exercise will help sedate excess liver qi and aid the smooth flow of qi, for which the liver is responsible.

4. Point Respiration: The hands remain one on top of the other, held in front of the liver. Concentrate the mind and focus your intention on the liver area and organ. Inhale and exhale through the nose. As you inhale, breathe into the liver. Exhale while lightly pressing or squeezing the area of the liver with the hands, imagining healing light radiating out of the liver as you press. Inhale and lift the hands away from the liver as you visualize white healing light flowing into the liver organ like a bellows. Repeat for 12 inhalations and exhalations. Close by leading the qi down into the lower dantian on an exhale.

5. End with Pulling Down the Heavens: When lowering the arms in front of the torso on the exhale, imagine the energy of the liver like water, melting and flowing down with the hands and filling the lower dantian. The qi is stored in the lower dantian so that the gathered energy will not be easily dispersed.

Lung Massage

1. Stand in Wuji posture and begin to breathe deeply. Relax the mind and visualize your body melting into the ground on the exhale.

2. Lung Regulation: Place both palms on the lungs, slightly higher than the breast area and below the clavicles (collar bones). Circle both hands out, down along the outsides of the breasts, in towards the midline, and back up the midline to the starting position. Repeat these circular rotations 12 times. Then massage 12 times using circles in the opposite direction: in and down the midline, and back up along the outsides of the breasts. The mind's focus should be on the lungs.

3. Point Respiration: With the hands at starting position, concentrate the mind and focus your intention on the lungs. Inhale and exhale through the nose. As you inhale, breathe into the lungs to fill each lung fully. Exhale while lightly pressing or squeezing the area of the chest where the hands are placed, imagining white healing light

radiating out of both lungs as you press. Inhale and lift the hands away from the lungs as you visualize healing light flowing into the lungs like a bellows. Repeat for 12 inhalations and exhalations. Close by leading the qi down into the lower dantian on an exhale. Patients with weak lung qi should concentrate their focus on filling the lungs with qi on the inhale, and feeling the cells of the lungs vibrate and glow with that qi on the exhale.

4.   End with Pulling Down the Heavens: When lowering the arms in front of the torso on the exhale, imagine the energy of the lungs like water, melting and flowing down with the hands and filling the lower dantian. The qi is stored in the lower dantian so that the gathered energy will not be easily dispersed.

Spleen and Stomach Massage

1.   Stand in Wuji posture and begin to breathe deeply. Relax the mind and visualize your body melting into the ground on the exhale.

2.   Spleen & Stomach Regulation: Place right hand over the stomach the left hand on top of the right hand. Massage in 12 circular rotations to the left in a clockwise direction, so that the circles are also over the spleen organ which is located to the left of the stomach. (Think of the stomach as being on the right side of the circle, and the spleen on the left side of the circle). Then perform 12 rotations in the opposite direction. When massaging, focus the mind on the digestive energy of the spleen and the stomach, imagining the qi flowing around those organs in accordance with the movements of the hands.

3.   Point Respiration: The hands remain one on top of the other, held slightly to the left of the stomach. Concentrate the mind and focus your intention on the spleen and stomach area. Inhale and exhale through the nose. As you inhale, breathe into the spleen and stomach. Exhale while lightly pressing or squeezing the area with the hands, imagining white healing light radiating out of the spleen and stomach area as you press. Inhale and lift the hands away as you visualize healing light flowing into the spleen and stomach organs like a bellows. Repeat for 12 inhalations and exhalations. Close by leading the qi down into the lower dantian on an exhale.

4.   End with Pulling Down the Heavens: When lowering the arms in front of the torso on the exhale, imagine the energy of the spleen and stomach like water, melting and flowing down with the hands and filling the lower dantian. The qi is stored in the lower dantian so that the gathered energy will not be easily dispersed.

Kidney Massage
1. Stand in Wuji posture and begin to breathe deeply. Relax the mind and visualize your body melting into the ground on the exhale.
2. Kidney Regulation: Place both palms on the low back below the ribcage. (Middle fingers should be over Urinary Bladder 23 at the level of the mingmen). Focus the mind on the kidneys. Vigorously rub both hands on the low back towards the spine and away from the spine to create warmth and heat in the low back area. Repeat 24-48 times.
3. Point Respiration: With the hands on the low back, concentrate the mind and focus your intention on the lungs. Exhale while lightly pressing or squeezing the area of the kidneys where the hands are placed, imagining white light radiating out of both kidneys as you press. Inhale and lift the hands away from the kidneys as you visualize healing light flowing into the kidneys, filling them like a bellows. Repeat for 12-36 breaths.
4. Place the right hand on the navel and the left on the center of the low back (mingmen). Use your intention to gather and consolidate the heat and qi in the kidneys and lower dantian. Breathe into and out of the area for 6-12 breaths.
5. End with Pulling Down the Heavens: When lowering the arms in front of the torso on the exhale, imagine the energy of the kidneys filling the lower dantian.

This exercise is excellent for tonifying the kidneys, and addresses the following disorders: impotence, premature ejaculation, lumbago, and pelvic inflammatory disease. Qigong and health practitioners should practice this exercise regularly, as it helps to increase their own qi, and qi projection when treating patients.

Qigong Self-Healing Acupoint Therapy
These exercises are performed towards the end of the qigong practice after the prescription exercises and before a closing exercise to end a session. Acupoint stimulation and gentle tapping disperse stagnation and blockages in the body and stimulate the flow of energy along the meridian channels.

The following is considered a complete set, and each exercise should be repeated from three to nine times before moving on to the next. Perform the exercises in the order presented from start to finish, or choose one or two that are appropriate.

1. **Ten Dragons Run Through the Forest:** Rub all ten fingers along the scalp from the front hairline over the head and to the neck. Visualize gathering and pulling out excess heat out of the head with the hands as they come to the neck.

2. **Rubbing the Ears:** Place left hand on left ear and right hand on right ear. Rub entire ear with thumb and pointer finger from bottom to top and top to bottom. Gently pull each ear away from head. Stimulates kidney qi and mental faculties. The ears have a direct neurological link with the brain and they are energetically connected to the kidneys.

3. **Rooting Qi from Chest to Abdomen:** Place left palm on center of chest at throat level and brush down the body's center line to below navel. Repeat with right palm, and continue to alternate hands as you visualize sinking and rooting the qi into the lower dantian. Calms anxiety and balances energy in upper and lower torso.

4. **Stimulating Large Intestine 4 (Tapping the Hands):** Place both hands in front of body and tap the dorsal aspect of the webbing between the thumb and pointer finger from each hand against the other. Promotes circulation and disperses pathogenic wind. Improves immunity.

5. **Stimulating Pericardium 6 (Tapping the Forearms):** Make a soft fist and tap the inside of the arm, approximately 3 finger-widths up from the wrist. Tap 9 times on left arm, and then 9 times on right arm. Regulates the qi and blood of the heart and stomach. Calms the heart.

6. **Stimulating Large Intestine 11 (Tapping the Elbows):** Continuing up the arm from Pericardium 6, tap the dorsal (lateral) aspect of the elbow fold of each arm 9 times. Dispels pathogenic qi, regulates the intestines, relaxes muscles, cools heat.

7. **Stimulating Heart 1 (Massaging the Armpits):** The right hand reaches under the left armpit and massages the area in 9 circular rotations, and then switch to the right armpit. Regulates heart qi and blood circulation.

8. **Rooting Qi from Chest to Abdomen:** Place left palm on center of chest at throat level and brush down the body's center line to below navel. Repeat with right palm, and continue to alternate hands as you visualize sinking and rooting the qi into the lower dantian. (Same as #3 above). Calms anxiety and balances energy in upper and lower torso.

9. **Stimulating the Gall Bladder Meridian (Dispersing Qi Down the Legs):** Make soft fists with each hand. Gently tap the buttocks and continue tapping down the sides of both legs simultaneously, along the lateral thighs, and down to just below the knees. Alleviates pain and tension in the thighs and legs. Disperses wind damp and cold.

10. **Stimulating the Lower Yin Meridians (Dispersing Qi from the Lower Legs):** With soft fists, continue tapping from below the outer knee area to the area below the inner knee. Continue to tap down the insides of the lower legs to the ankles. Regulates spleen, kidney, and liver meridians, strengthens the lower jiao.

11. **Stimulating Kidney 1 (Dropping the Heels):** With the knees slightly bent, quickly rise on to the toes and then fall on both heels, and repeat in quick succession. To end, shake out the back to disperse tension. Tonifies kidneys, calms the mind, disperses pathogenic and stagnant qi into the ground.

12. **Closing (Sealing the Lower Dantian)** : Place one palm on the lower abdomen and the other palm on top of that hand. Circle 12 times counter clockwise, and then 12 times clockwise. Rest the hands just below the navel and visualize the body's energy pooling in the lower dantian.

EXERCISE PRESCRIPTIONS FOR PARTICULAR ORGAN IMBALANCES

LIVER AND GALLBLADDER DISORDERS

Rx for Tonifying the Liver

Taking in the Green Qi Meditation

This powerful meditation makes use of the energetic attributes of color. As mentioned previously, five element theory assigns a color to each organ system, and that color strengthens deficiency in the organ it targets. Green is the color associated with the liver and gall bladder.

1. Stand in Wuji posture. (Alternatively, you may sit in a chair or lie on your back). Relax the whole body and quiet the mind. Breathe deeply and naturally. Place the tongue where the upper teeth meet the roof of the mouth.

2. Visualize green energy in front of you, like a mist or a pulsating, vibrating green orb. To aid the visualization, picture trees and the feeling of being in a forest. You may also perform this exercise amongst trees to enhance the wood element aspect of the meditation.

3. Inhale green light energy through the nose and down into the liver organ. Feel the area vibrate with the green color.

4. As you exhale through the mouth, visualize dark, pathogenic qi leaving the liver via the mouth as a black cloud. While the darkness leaves, the clean, bright green color remains in the liver.

5. With each inhale, the liver retains more clean energy and glows brighter with vitality.

6. With each exhale, the dark cloud becomes lighter and lighter.

7. Inhale and exhale in this manner for approximately five minutes.

8. To close, breathe in the color green through the nose, and imagine it filling the entire mouth. On the exhale (through the nose), send the green qi down to the liver, and then into the abdomen to fill the lower dantian. Repeat 8 times.

Rx for Dispersing Liver Qi Stagnation and/or Gall Bladder Excess Conditions

Descending the Yang and Ascending the Yin Technique

This exercise activates the flow of qi in the lower body channels. It lowers stagnant qi from the body into the earth, and raises clean qi up the yin meridians to the lower and middle dantian. Repeat for a total of nine times on each leg, or practice for 10 minutes, twice a day.

1. Stand in Wuji posture. Place the palms on the lower abdomen. Visualize qi gathering beneath your palms.
2. Turn the upper torso towards the left by twisting from the waist, and brush both palms to the left hip and down the lateral aspect of the left thigh, along the gall bladder channel. Visualize your hands gathering and pushing qi down the leg and into the earth. Continue pushing both hands down the leg until you reach the ankle (the lateral malleolus).
3. Shift the hands to the inside of the ankle (medial malleolus), and pull earthly qi up the inside of the left leg, which is along the three leg yin channels.
4. Continue to pull earth qi up along the inside of the thigh, through the lower dantian, and into the middle dantian. Visualize the earth qi filling and vitalizing the area of the liver and gall bladder.
5. Gather the energy from the liver and gall bladder and turn the upper torso to the right by twisting from the waist.
6. Descend the qi with the palms along the lateral aspect of the right leg. Continue pushing the qi from the liver and gall bladder down the leg and into the earth.
7. When the hands reach the ankle, shift them to the inner ankle and pull qi from the earth up the inside of the right leg.
8. Continue up the right leg and pull the qi through the lower dantian and into the middle dantian. Feel it fill the area of the liver and gall bladder. Repeat the exercise, pushing and gathering the qi down the left leg.
9. End by sinking the qi into the lower dantian. Remain in Wuji for a few breaths.

After completing Descending the Yang and Ascending the Yin, perform the Liver Massage exercise (See Organ Self Massage section). Vocalize the sound "shu" on the exhale throughout the exercise. Repeat for 36 breaths.

Rx for Liver Fire or Liver Yang Rising

Liver fire and liver fire rising are often associated with hypertension, migraines, tension headaches, and/or a tendency to be excessively warm.

Anti-hypertensive Breathing Technique

Hypertensives often breathe only into the upper areas of the lung. On the inhale, their shoulders and upper chest will rise, but the remainder of the body is still. Breathing in this way causes an accumulation of qi and tension in the upper body, particularly around the heart and neck. The style of breathing used to help alleviate high blood pressure and calm the nerves is called "natural breathing," or "fetal breathing." It is how babies breathe when they are infants, and how we all breathed before we consciously experienced stress in our lives. It sinks the qi from the upper body into the lower body, and will lower blood pressure while performed. Changes in diet and lifestyle are necessary to maximize the benefits of this exercise.

1. Sit in a chair or stand in Wuji posture. Relax the body and quiet the mind.
2. Inhale through the nose as you purposefully stick the abdomen (belly) out. Focus on breathing into the abdomen, filling the lungs from the bottom to the top. Keep the shoulders and neck relaxed.
3. Exhale through the nose as you pull the abdomen in. Exhale slowly and deeply from the lower lungs to the top, until the lungs are empty.
4. Repeat for 10 minutes, two times a day if possible. Make sure the muscles remain relaxed and the breath is deep and slow.

Water Visualization

This exercise is extremely simple yet effective. Sit in a chair. Inhale a deep, relaxed breath into the lower abdomen. Exhale and imagine the feeling of warm or even slightly cool water being gently poured over the head. Feel it flow down the front, back and sides of the body, taking with it all tension and heat. Visualize your body being coated with and bathed by the water until the water reaches your feet and saturates the ground around you. Practice this three times a day, 36 breaths each time.

You can add the exercise of rubbing the liver area (hypochrondrium) with both hands and toning the sound "shu" to purge excess heat from the liver, or use the following exercise.

Pulling Down Heavens with Shu Sound

1. Stand in Wuji posture.
2. Begin Pulling Down Heavens, but make the inhale and the rising of the hands quicker than usual.
3. Exhale very slowly and consciously, and vocalize the "shu" sound with a descending tone while the hands slowly lower down the front of the body.
4. Repeat 36 times, 2 times a day.

HEART DISORDERS

Rx for Tonifying the Heart and Heart Blood

Taking in the Red Qi Meditation

This powerful meditation makes use of the energetic attributes of color. Five element theory assigns a color to each organ system, and that color strengthens deficiency in the organ it targets. Red is the color associated with the heart, the blood, and the small intestines. Taking in the Red Meditation is excellent for coronary heart disease, angina, arrhythmia, rheumatic heart disease, palpitations, and blood-deficiency related insomnia.

Caveat: If a person has a deficient heart (heart qi deficiency) but also suffers from an excess heat condition, he or she should visualize the color pink rather than red.

1. Stand in Wuji posture. (Alternatively, you may sit in a chair or lie on your back). Relax the whole body and quiet the mind. Breathe deeply and naturally. Place the tongue where the upper teeth meet the roof of the mouth.
2. Visualize red energy in front of you, like a mist or a pulsating, vibrating red orb. To aid the visualization, picture a bright red sunrise or sunset and the feeling of being in its presence. You may also perform this exercise at sunrise to enhance the fire element aspect of the meditation.
3. Inhale red light energy through the nose and down into the heart organ. Feel the area vibrate with the red color.
4. As you exhale through the mouth, visualize dark, pathogenic qi leaving the heart via the mouth as a black cloud. While the darkness leaves, the clean, bright red color remains in the heart.
5. With each inhale, the heart retains more clean energy and glows brighter with vitality.
6. With each exhale, the dark cloud becomes lighter and lighter.
7. Inhale and exhale in this manner for approximately five minutes.
8. To close, breathe in the color red through the nose, and imagine it filling the entire mouth. On the exhale (through the nose), send the red qi down to the heart, and then into the abdomen to fill the lower dantian and connect with the kidneys. Repeat 7 to 14 times.

RX for Purging the Heart

This exercise is used for excess heat or anxiety trapped in the heart or chest area.

1. Stand in Wuji posture. Relax the body and quiet the mind.
2. Place the tongue in the fire position, which is behind the upper teeth where they meet the roof of the mouth.

3. Place one hand over the heart (on the left side of the chest) and the other hand over the first hand. Alternatively, you can place the hands over the center of the chest if it feels more appropriate.
4. Inhale deeply and circle the hands clockwise over the heart or center of the chest to stimulate the tissues. Connect your intention to the heart.
5. Exhale the sound "ha", as you pull the hands away from the chest. Imagine that your palms are like magnets, pulling the heat or anxiety out as they lift off the chest.
6. Repeat for 6 to 12 breaths

RX for Weak or Elderly Patients with Hypertension

This exercise can be performed either lying supine or sitting in a chair. The "zheng" sound, (pronounced "jang"), targets the blood and blood vessels directly. This exercise is also useful for clearing heat from the blood of people who do not have hypertension.

1. Lie supine with a pillow under the head, or sit upright in a chair.
2. Imagine that you are floating in warm water.
3. Inhale deeply and then exhale the "zheng" sound.
4. As you exhale, feel or imagine the "zheng" sound vibrate the body's tissues from the top of the head downwards, through the chest and abdomen, down the legs, and out the feet.
5. Repeat for several minutes and then end with a focus on the bottoms of the feet (Kidney 1 points).

SPLEEN AND STOMACH DIGESTIVE DISORDERS

RX for Tonifying the Spleen

Taking in the Yellow Qi

This powerful meditation makes use of the energetic attributes of color. Five element theory assigns a color to each organ system, and that color strengthens deficiency in the organ it targets. Yellow is the color associated with the spleen and stomach, the two organs most responsible for strong digestion. Taking in the Yellow Meditation is excellent for chronic gas, bloating, diarrhea, constipation, colitis, and general digestive weakness.

1. Stand in Wuji posture. (Alternatively, you may sit in a chair or lie on your back). Relax the whole body and quiet the mind. Breathe deeply and naturally.
2. Visualize yellow energy in front of you, like a mist or a pulsating, vibrating yellow orb. To aid the visualization, picture a patch of bright yellow flowers and the feeling of being in its presence.

3. Inhale yellow light energy through the nose and down into the stomach and spleen organs (the spleen is located to the left of the stomach). Feel the area vibrate with the yellow color.

4. As you exhale through the mouth, visualize dark, turbid, damp pathogenic qi leaving the spleen and stomach via the mouth as a moist black cloud. While the darkness leaves, the clean, bright yellow color remains in the spleen and stomach.

5. With each inhale, the digestive organs retain more clean energy and glow brighter with vitality.

6. With each exhale, the dark cloud becomes lighter and lighter.

7. Inhale and exhale in this manner for approximately five minutes.

8. To close, breathe in the color yellow through the nose, and imagine it filling the entire mouth. On the exhale (through the nose), send the yellow qi to the stomach area (Ren 12), down to the lower dantian, and then feel it spread out to the four limbs, the skin, and the hair. Repeat 7 to 14 times.

RX for Purging the Spleen

Dredging the Spleen and Stomach

The following exercise stimulates the spleen and stomach channels, and purges dampness and heat from the spleen and stomach organs. This exercise is excellent for sluggish digestion, ulcers, and acid reflux. Practice this exercise twice a day.

1. Stand in Wuji posture. Relax every muscle in the body from head to toe. Quiet the mind and breathe deeply and naturally.

2. Allow the arms to hang loosely as you twist the upper body at the waist to the left side. At the same time, the arms swing in front of the body to the right side (the opposite direction of the torso), gently hitting the body where they land.

3. Twist from the waist to the right as the arms float in front of the body to the left and land against the waist area.

4. Be sure that the head follows the twist of the upper body. The twist should be deep but comfortable. The mind should be focused on the heels.

5. Repeat from one side to the other until you feel tension released from the whole body.

6. Place one palm over the other and place the bottom palm over the stomach on the upper abdomen.

7. Rub clockwise for three to six circles as you inhale. Focus the mind on the stomach.

8. Sound the "hu" sound on the exhale as you lift the palms gently away from the body. Visualize the palms as magnets, pulling all tension and stagnation out of the stomach.

9. Repeat steps 7 and 8 for five minutes.
10. To close, visualize the qi of the spleen and stomach lower and settle into the lower dantian.

Rx to Improve Digestive Flow

Descending and Ascending Earth Qi

This exercise stimulates the flow of qi in the spleen and stomach channels, and prepares the spleen and stomach organs for tonification. It pulls earth qi into the body while sinking rebellious stomach qi (stomach qi that is rising instead of sinking). Excellent for nausea, heartburn, irritable bowel, and stagnant digestion.

1. Stand in Wuji posture. Relax every muscle of the body and quiet the mind. Breathe naturally and deeply.
2. Place both palms on the upper abdomen approximately level with the stomach (Ren 12), with fingertips slightly facing each other.
3. Gather the energy of the stomach into each hand, visualizing the stomach energy as two vibrating yellow balls of light.
4. Pull the two balls of qi out to the sides of the torso and down past the waist. The left hand pulls down the left side of the body, and the right hand pulls down the right side of the body.
5. Continue to push the yellow qi down the lateral aspects of the legs, past the thighs and knees, to the ankles. Visualize pushing the qi past the ankles and into the ground.
6. Shift the palms over the feet to the insides of the ankles, and visualize earth energy gathering up from the earth and into your hands.
7. Pull the earth energy up the insides of the legs. Continue pulling up past the inner thighs and into the stomach. Feel the energy fill and energize the stomach.
8. Repeat 18 times.
9. To close, visualize the qi from the stomach lower and sink into the lower dantian.

Swaying the Arms While Beating and Drumming the Qi:

This exercise stimulates and massages the five yang organs. It specifically strengthens the peristaltic action of the digestive system and stimulates the autonomic nervous system. This exercise regulates digestion, making it appropriate for people with spastic colon, colitis, irritable bowel, diarrhea and/or constipation, and Crohn's disease. Do not eat within one hour prior to practicing.

1. Stand in Wuji posture with legs wider than shoulders' distance apart.
2. Inhale into the abdomen and swing the arms forward and up to the height of the armpits with palms down.

3. While still inhaling, drop the elbows and pull the hands in towards the body with palms parallel to the ground. (Like a dog begging). The hands come in towards the body at the approximate height of the armpits. Steps 2 and 3 are performed as one flowing move.
4. Exhale, pull in the abdomen, and swing the arms forward and down until they are pressing backwards with palms facing back.
5. Lift arms and begin again. The pace should be a quick but comfortable flow.
6. When inhaling, fill the abdomen and stick out the belly. When exhaling, contract the abdomen and visualize the qi flow from the navel down to the perineum, to the low back (mingmen). On the subsequent inhale, feel the qi flow back towards the navel, filling the lower abdomen. The anal sphincter should be held gently closed throughout the exercise.
7. Repeat for 50 to 250 breaths.

LUNG DISORDERS

Rx for Tonifying the Lungs

Taking in the White Qi Meditation

This powerful meditation makes use of the energetic attributes of color. Five element theory assigns a color to each organ system, and that color strengthens deficiency in the organ it targets. White is the color associated with the lungs and large intestine. Taking in the White Meditation is excellent for chronic asthma, cough, emphysema, chronic bronchitis, dyspnea, and weak lung qi in general.

1. Stand in Wuji posture. (Alternatively, you may sit in a chair or lie on your back). Relax the whole body and quiet the mind. Breathe deeply and naturally.
2. Visualize white energy in front of you, like a mist or a pulsating, vibrating white orb. To aid the visualization, picture a bright full moon and the feeling of being in its presence.
3. Inhale white light energy through the nose and down into the lungs. Fill each lung entirely. Feel the lungs vibrate with the white color.
4. As you exhale through the mouth, visualize dark, turbid, pathogenic qi leaving the lungs via the mouth as a black cloud. While the darkness leaves, the clean, bright white color remains in the lungs.
5. With each inhale, the lungs retain more clean energy and glow brighter with vitality.
6. With each exhale, the dark cloud becomes lighter and lighter.
7. Inhale and exhale in this manner for approximately five minutes.

8. To close, breathe in the color white through the nose, and imagine it filling the entire mouth. On the exhale (through the nose), send the white qi to the depths of the lungs, down to the lower dantian, and then feel it spread out to the four limbs, the skin, and the hair. Repeat 9 to 18 times.

Rx for Purging the Lungs

This exercise helps drain stagnation from the lungs. It is used for excess conditions such as heat trapped in the lungs, phlegm dampness, and asthma.

1. Place the hands on the chest below the collar bones. Focus your attention on the lungs.
2. Inhale as fully as possible from the bottom of the lungs to the top.
3. Exhale the sound "ssss" as the hands circle out (while touching the chest) towards the sides of the body, down along the outsides of the breasts, and back in and up the centerline.
4. Repeat for 12 to 24 breaths.

Rx for Regulating the Lungs and Conducting the Qi

This exercise is practiced after the lungs have been tonified or purged. It is a regulating exercise that helps improve breath capacity and the circulation of lung qi.

1. Sit with the legs crossed on either the floor, a bed, a couch, or another suitable piece of furniture.
2. Place the hands directly down on the sides of the body, with palms resting on the floor's surface.
3. Inhale through the nose, pressing the palms into the floor, and arching the spine backwards. The chest should be pressed forwards and the breath should fill the lungs completely.
4. Pause briefly before exhaling.
5. Exhale through the nose, drawing the chest in and leaning slightly forward. Exhale until the lungs are empty.
6. Repeat 4 to 9 times.
7. Place the palms on the knees and sit with a straight spine.
8. Inhale through the nose as you turn the torso and head to the left.
9. Turn to center, lean slightly forward, and exhale through the nose. Return to a straight spine.
10. Inhale as you turn the torso and head to the right.
11. Turn to center, lean slightly forward, and exhale through the nose.
12. Always inhale while turning, and exhale while facing forward.
13. Repeat 4 to 9 times.

Rx for the Common Head Cold

The following self-massage technique purges pathogenic wind from the gall bladder channels on the head. Used when a common cold is lodged in the head, leading to headache, foggy thinking, and neck and shoulder tightness.

Ten Dragons Run Through the Forest
1. Place all of the fingertips at the front hairline, with the left hand on the left of the midline, and the right hand on the right of the midline.
2. Fingertips should be pointing towards the back of the head.
3. Rub all ten fingers along the scalp from the front hairline over the head and down to the neck.
4. Visualize the hands gathering and pulling wind out of the head and neck, continuing down to the shoulders.
5. Once the hands reach the shoulders, visualize gathering the qi in each hand and then tossing it down into the earth.
6. Once you have the motion, try to inhale as the hands move from the head to the shoulders, and exhale as you toss the pathogenic qi.
7. Repeat 24 to 50 times.

Rx for Chronic Asthma, Lung Qi Deficiency, and Bronchitis

Daoist Lung Tonification and Regulation Exercise
1. Place the arms in front of the body at shoulder level with palms facing down. The elbows should be bent so that the fingertips are diagonally pointing towards each other, and the arms should feel as if resting on water. Relax the shoulders.
2. Inhale and bring the arms out to the sides, leading with the elbows. Squeeze the shoulder blades together while keeping the shoulders relaxed.
3. Turn the palms up, exhale, and bring the arms back towards starting position with the palms up. As the hands reach the starting position, turn the palms down.
4. Repeat 20 times, twice a day. You can add the color white on the inhale, and/or the "shh" sound on the exhale if desired.

RX for Sinusitis and Sinus Pain

Bathing & Kneading the Nose
1. Rub the outer sides of the thumbs together until they become warm or hot.
2. Place the sides of the thumbs on both sides of the nose.
3. Gently rub up and down using the entire side of each thumb for 10 breaths.

4. Place the tips of the middle fingers on both sides of the nose, in the depression lateral to the nostrils (Large Intestine 20).
5. Rub in small circles, using strong pressure.
6. Continue this method laterally out and across the cheeks, to the depression below and in line with the pupils of the eyes (Stomach 3).
7. Slowly work your way back and then rub up along the sides of the nose to the eyes.
8. Repeat 10 times.

KIDNEY AND REPRODUCTIVE DISORDERS

RX for Tonifying the Kidneys

Taking in the Blue Qi Meditation

This powerful meditation makes use of the energetic attributes of color. Five element theory assigns a color to each organ system, and that color strengthens deficiency in the organ it targets. Dark blue is the color associated with the kidneys, urinary bladder, bones, bone marrow, and the brain. Taking in the Blue Qi Meditation is excellent for tonifying the kidneys and urinary bladder, and strengthens the bones in cases of osteopoenia and osteoporosis.

1. Stand in Wuji posture. (Alternatively, you may sit in a chair or lie on your back). Relax the whole body and quiet the mind. Breathe deeply and naturally. Place the tongue where the upper teeth meet the roof of the mouth.
2. Visualize dark, deep blue energy in front of you, like a mist or a pulsating, vibrating blue orb. To aid the visualization, picture a dark blue, deep ocean and the feeling of being in its presence. You may also perform this exercise at a lake, river, or the ocean to enhance the water element aspect of the meditation.
3. Inhale blue light energy through the nose and down into the kidney organs. Feel the area of the low back vibrate with the dark blue color.
4. As you exhale through the mouth, visualize dark, pathogenic qi leaving the low back and kidney area via the mouth as a black cloud. While the darkness leaves, the clean, bright blue color remains in the kidneys.
5. With each inhale, the kidneys retain more clean energy and glow brighter with vitality.
6. With each exhale, the dark cloud becomes lighter and lighter.
7. Inhale and exhale in this manner for approximately five minutes.
8. To close, breathe in the color blue through the nose, and imagine it filling the entire mouth. On the exhale (through the nose), send the blue qi down into the kidneys, and then into the abdomen to fill the lower dantian. Repeat 6 to 12 times.

Rx for Tinnitus and Deafness

Beating the Heavenly Drum and Pressing the Ears

Chinese medicine associates the ears with the kidneys, as the ears are the sensory "openings" or "orifices" of the kidneys. The energy and function of the ears is directly related to kidney qi. Tinnitus and deafness can arise from weak kidney qi or jing, or excess liver qi rising to the ears. Therefore, the kidneys should first be strengthened, and/or the liver sedated before practicing this exercise. This exercise balances the air pressure in the eustachian tubes and ear canals, helps prevent vertigo, dispels accumulated qi from the back of the head, and stimulates the pineal gland. In addition, it stimulates kidney qi and hearing.

1. Begin by rubbing the palms together to warm the hands.
2. Stand in Wuji posture, but place the feet into a wider stance for balance.
3. Place the palms over the ears, with the fingers touching at the back of the head just above the neck (the area of Du 16 & Urinary Bladder 9, otherwise known as the occipital protuberance or "jade pillow").
4. Press the palms into the ears and rest the left index fingertip over the right index fingertip. Close the eyes.
5. Lift the right index finger up so that the left index finger makes a thump sound onto the back of the head.
6. Repeat the thumping sound, alternating the right and left index fingers. The thump should be rhythmic, like a heart beat.
7. Continue for 36 repetitions.
8. Bend forward, keeping the hands in place. Clench the jaws together slightly and comfortably.
9. Exhale while bending forward, and bring the head as close to between the legs as possible.
10. Hold the breath and look through the legs to the area behind the body.
11. Raise the body up and inhale before beginning the series again from step 1.
12. Repeat the entire sequence up to 14 times.

Pressing the Ears: After completing the Beating the Heavenly Drum exercise, press the palms into the ears to create a gentle suction. Pull the palms out and off the ears. Repeat 9 times.

Rx for Back Pain and Tightness

Opening, Collecting and Moving the Qi (Stretching the Spine)

This exercise stretches and loosens the spinal vertebrae and facilitates energy flow through the patient's spine and Du channel. It stimulates the central nervous system and cerebral spinal fluid. In addition, it stretches the connective tissues, frees adhesions, and enhances the elasticity and compressibility of the tendons, ligaments, and joints. If you encounter any pain or limitations, honor them and do not push past them. Find your comfort zone and stay within it.

1. Inhale as you raise both hands above the head. Imagine energy (like a rushing river) flowing up from the feet, filling the legs, hips, waist, chest, arms, and head. Every square inch of the body is absorbing and being saturated with earth energy. When the entire body is completely full, the hands should still be positioned above the head as if you were going to dive into a pool.
2. Exhale and feel the hands getting very heavy. The heaviness pulls the hands forward and then slowly starts to pull the body over. Slowly bend the head forward and feel the cervical vertebrae stretch. Let the hands pull the arms, which in turn pull the shoulders and torso, followed by bending at the waist. The purpose of this movement is to feel each vertebra of the spine stretch sequentially so that a rippling effect descends down the spine.
3. As you exhale while bending over, imagine the energy melting away from the entire body (like ice melting into water) slowly dissolving and rushing down through the feet and out into the ground.
4. Once completely bent over, imagine picking up a very large ball, so that the elbows are slightly pointed towards each other and the hands are palms up. Inhale, bend the knees, and slowly stand up. While standing up, reverse the rippling of the spine from coccyx, sacrum, and lower lumbar vertebrae to base of skull. The head should be the last body part to become vertical.
5. Inhale while raising the body and until you have both arms over your head.
6. Exhale as the body descends.
7. Repeat for 5-10 minutes.

Rx for Impotence

Impotence, from a Chinese medicine viewpoint, is often related to the strength of the kidney yang. When the kidney yang is weak, the sex drive and/or the strength of erections is diminished. Often there are also psychological factors influencing sexual function. If this is the case, the practitioner should include meditations that calm the heart and spirit. Deep breathing meditations can be beneficial for relieving performance anxiety, fear, and over-excitement.

Deer Exercise for Increasing Body's Jing

This exercise brings energy to the prostate, penis and testicles. It helps improve quality and quantity of sperm and relieves impotence.

1. Sit on the edge of a chair. Rub the palms together to create heat.
2. Cup the testicles with the right hand so that the palm completely covers them with slight pressure.

3. The left hand is placed on the lower dantian below the navel. The left hand rubs the lower abdomen in clockwise circles. Circle 81 times. Concentrate on the heat and qi filling the lower dantian and genital area.

4. The hands are then rubbed together again. Switch hands and cup the testicles with the left hand while placing the right hand on the lower dantian.

5. The right hand circles the lower abdomen 81 times in a counter-clockwise direction. Focus on the heat and qi filling the lower dantian and genital area.

6. Once the circles on the abdomen are completed, inhale while tightening and drawing up the anal muscles. Feel the qi being drawn up the rectum and prostate area, filling the lower dantian.

7. Hold the breath as long as possible. Exhale, release the muscles and relax.

8. This should be repeated for 25 breaths, and over time the practitioner should work up to 250 breaths.

MISCELLANEOUS DISORDERS

Rx for Headaches & Migraines

Meditation for Headache Prevention

This exercise should be practiced daily to prevent the onset of headaches. The practitioner focuses on draining the qi, blood, and heat out of the head and down the extremities. This can be practiced from a sitting, reclining, or lying down posture.

1. Close the eyes. Relax and quiet the mind. Take a few deep breaths.

2. Imagine that it is summertime, and that you are at the beach. Take a minute to create that visualization.

3. Focus your attention on your arms and hands. Imagine them becoming warmer and warmer, as if the sun is beating down on them.

4. Continue to feel the sun beating down on the arms and hands until they feel hot. Visualize the blood and energy of the head being pulled towards the hands.

5. Feel your face becoming cooler as the pressure and pain melt down the neck, past the shoulders, through the arms, and out the hands.

6. If you wish, you can add the legs and feet by feeling them become warm as the energy from the head drains out and down the legs and feet as well as the hands.

Rx for Insomnia

This exercise should be repeated nightly just before going to sleep. Practice this exercise while sitting at the edge of the bed.

1. Slap your hands together and rub them until they become warm.

2. Close the eyes and place both hands on the low back over the kidneys at waist level. Place your intention on the kidneys.
3. Massage by rubbing the low back with both hands towards and away from the spine 36 times.
4. With the hands on the low back, inhale the heat from the low back into the kidneys. Inhale and exhale the heat into the kidneys for three breaths.
5. Repeat steps 3 and 4.
6. After the final inhale and exhale, place one hand on the lower dantian below the navel and leave one hand on the mingmen. Inhale the heat from the back of the body into the front of the body and the lower dantian. Repeat for a total of three breaths.
7. Put the right leg (ankle) over the left knee. Rub the bottom of the right foot (over the Kidney 1 point) with left hand 100 times back and forth towards the toes. Visualize the energy descending from the leg into the foot.
8. Switch legs and place the left leg (ankle) over the right knee. Rub the bottom of the left foot 100 times while visualizing the energy of the leg descend into the foot.

Rx for Menstrual Disorders & Fertility

Turning and Winding the Belt Vessel
   The following exercise stimulates the energy moving within the Dai channel, also known as the belt vessel. The Dai channel is a meridian that circles the waist. It is often used to treat menstrual disorders and fertility difficulties. If there are menstrual problems such as cramping, PMS, and distention pain, the practitioner should add exercises that soothe the liver. If there is blood or kidney deficiency, exercises that tonify blood and kidneys should be added.

1. Stand in Wuji posture. Practice abdominal breathing and gently close the anal sphincter. Place both hands over the right kidney.
2. Raise both hands out to the right side of the body with the palms facing down. The hands should be approximately level with the waist.
3. Twisting from the waist, circle both hands to the left towards the front of the body as if they are resting on or skimming the surface of a lake.
4. Continue to circle the arms around the front of the body to the left until you cannot twist further. Inhale when the hands are circling in front of the body. Focus the mind on absorbing energy from the earth into the hands, and from the hands into the lower dantian. The hands should come to rest on the low back over the left kidney.
5. Take both palms and rub them along the path of the waist from the left kidney, past the navel, and back to the right kidney. Exhale as the hands

brush across the waist. Focus the mind on consolidating the qi in the lower dantian.

6.   Repeat the circles 36 times.

7.   Begin again, this time with the hands over the left kidney and circle the hands out towards the right. When the hands reach the right kidney, they brush across the waist back to the left kidney. Repeat from this side 36 times.

Rx for Spiritual and Emotional Development

Microcosmic Orbit Fire Cycle

This exercise calms and roots the mind as it fuses the body's main yang channel (the Du channel), with the body's main yin channel (the Ren channel). This will aid the discharge of toxic emotions from the body, and allow the practitioner better access to his or her yuan shen, or original spirit.

1.   Sit in meditation posture, or stand in Wuji posture with hands held facing the lower abdomen.

2.   Place the tongue on the roof of the mouth behind the upper teeth. Gently close the anal sphincter.

3.   Visualize qi like a red neon light rising up the back along the spine.

4.   Continue to feel the red qi travel over the head, down the face, and down the front of the body's center line.

5.   The red neon light continues down past the abdomen, genitals, perineum, and to the back, where it will continue to ascend.

6.   Inhale as the qi is pulled up the back to the top of the head.

7.   Exhale as the qi descends the front of the body to the perineum.

8.   Continue this practice for 20 minutes a day.

BIBLIOGRAPHY

Johnson, Jerry Alan, *The Essence of Internal Martial Arts Volume II*, Ching Lien Healing Arts Center, Pacific Grove, California, 1994.

Johnson, Jerry Alan, *Chinese Medical Qigong Therapy: A Comprehensive Clinical Text*, International Institute of Medical Qigong, Pacific Grove, California, 2000. (With permission, this book formed the basis for most of the content contained herein).

Oschman, James, *Energy Medicine in Therapeutics and Human Performance*, Elsevier Science, Philadelphia Pennsylvania, 2003.

Seem, Mark, with Kaplan, Joan, *Bodymind Energetics*, Healing Arts Press, Rochester, Vermont, 1989.

INDEX

Printed in the United States
84389LV00003B/225/A

9 781425 707149